Working
Wonders

Working Wonders

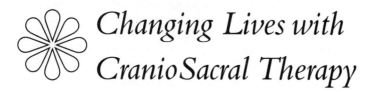 *Changing Lives with CranioSacral Therapy*

Case Studies from Practitioners of CST

Edited by
The Upledger Institute

Foreword by John E. Upledger, DO, OMM

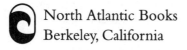

North Atlantic Books
Berkeley, California

UI Enterprises
Palm Beach Gardens, Florida

Published by   and
North Atlantic Books   UI Enterprises
P.O. Box 12327   11211 Prosperity Farms Road, Ste D-325
Berkeley, California 94712   Palm Beach Gardens, Florida 33410

Cover photo by C. J. Walker
Cover and book design by Paula Morrison
Printed in the United States of America
Distributed to the book trade by Publishers Group West

Working Wonders: Changing Lives with CranioSacral Therapy is sponsored by the Society for the Study of Native Arts and Sciences, a nonprofit educational corporation whose goals are to develop an educational and crosscultural perspective linking various scientific, social, and artistic fields; to nurture a holistic view of arts, sciences, humanities, and healing; and to publish and distribute literature on the relationship of mind, body, and nature.

North Atlantic Books' publications are available through most bookstores. For further information, call 800-337-2665 or visit our website at www.northatlanticbooks.com. Substantial discounts on bulk quantities are available to corporations, professional associations, and other organizations. For details and discount information, contact our special sales department.

Library of Congress Cataloging-in-Publication Data

Working wonders : changing lives with craniosacral therapy / by the Upledger Institute.
        p. ; cm.
    Summary: "A compilation of stories by practitioners of CranioSacral Therapy from around the world telling how the therapy made a difference in clients' lives. It includes cases involving children, adults, and animals"—Provided by publisher.
    ISBN 1-55643-605-X (pbk.)
    1. Craniosacral therapy.
    [DNLM: 1. Manipulation, Osteopathic—methods—Personal Narratives. 2. Massage—methods—Personal Narratives. 3. Complementary Therapies—Personal Narratives. 4. Manipulation, Osteopathic—veterinary—Personal Narratives. 5. Massage—veterinary—Personal Narratives.] I. Upledger Institute.
    RZ399.C73W675 2005
    615.8'2—dc22
                                        2005004304

    1 2 3 4 5 6 7 8 9 MALLOY 10 09 08 07 06 05

In commemoration of The Upledger Institute's twentieth anniversary in 2005.

This book is dedicated to the tens of thousands of CranioSacral Therapy practitioners around the world who have embraced the practice of CranioSacral Therapy, and to the incalculable number of patients who continue to inspire this work on a daily basis.

Table of Contents

CranioSacral Therapy and Adults

CranioSacral Therapy and Animals

Foreword

It is with great pleasure that I write the foreword to this collection of CranioSacral Therapy case histories. Over the years I have come to believe in the validity of clinical outcomes over scientific studies as support for various diagnostic and therapeutic modalities. In reading these stories, I believe you will see why. It is hard to dispute the evidence of actual changed lives. I have seen people with stroke syndromes recover in one CranioSacral Therapy session, people with long-time speech deficits normalize, blood pressures normalize, atrial fibrillations of several years disappear, central sleep apneas disappear, TMJ problems abate, and an Olympic diver return to training after a six-month lay-off secondary to vertigo. She traveled the country looking for relief from "scientifically qualified" treatment methods. After all else failed she came to see me. Ten treatments later she resumed her training *sans* vertigo and went on to win a bronze medal in the Atlanta games.

Still there are those who would discount the merit of CranioSacral Therapy based on the lack of "scientific" evidence. To them I offer one of my favorite quotes: "Absence of proof is not proof of absence" (William Cowper).

When you see newborns' heads reshape, colic disappear, seizures stop, medications discontinued, even children with congenital central hypoventilation syndrome obviate the need for breathing machines, you begin to believe your eyes, and the "double-blind study" becomes much less important.

For those who require it, however, substantiating research certainly exists. In fact, there is probably more solid evidence that supports CranioSacral Therapy and its uses than there is for the efficacy of coronary bypass surgery.

I first observed the rhythmical motion of the intact dura mater at mid-cervical level (a.k.a. the functioning craniosacral system) during a surgical procedure in 1972. This piqued my curiosity and began what would become years of laboratory and clinical research to understand its implications, an effort that has been widely supported in the field.

For eight and a half years I worked as a clinician-researcher in the Department of Biomechanics at Michigan State University with a team that included biophysicists, neurophysiologists, and bioengineers. Our work in both the laboratory and the clinic explored the therapeutic potentials of CranioSacral Therapy on everyone from newborns to the elderly, in both humans and primates.

My research continued during five years on the American Osteopathic Association's Bureau of Research and two years on the first Alternative Medicine Program Advisory Panel at the National Institutes of Health. Not long ago I received a letter from a prominent neurosurgeon in Switzerland who is highly regarded throughout Europe. After acknowledging the science I have used to understand the workings of the craniosacral system, he went on to note wonderful post-operative progress on a Swiss brain-surgery patient we shared. He said that he had performed twenty thousand surgeries during his extended career and had witnessed the rhythmical wave of the cerebrospinal fluid as I described it in my writings in at least half of those cases.

Through these and countless other experiences over the years, I have come to recognize the craniosacral system as highly sophisticated, extremely subtle, and very influential in its impact upon total body psychophysiology. The craniosacral system stops, starts, and modifies its functioning as it deems necessary to effectively control its various contributions to the lifehood of the body it resides in.

As remarkable and valuable as all this evidence is, however, what I keep coming back to is the conviction that what is really important in clinical practice is how the patient fares in response to what we do as therapists. CranioSacral Therapy recognizes that no two people are exactly alike; that each treatment protocol is dictated by the wisdom of a person's own body; and that no two sessions are alike.

As therapists we can be proud that the work we are performing and the compassionate care we are providing are improving the lives of people in need—many of whom had given up hope of ever finding relief or any measure of "quality" of life. That's why I prefer to believe my eyes, and the eyes of the CranioSacral Therapists in this book, over any scientific studies. Let's continue to have the courage to step beyond the bounds of conventional wisdom and trust the positive outcomes we are seeing.

—*John E. Upledger, DO, OMM*

CranioSacral Therapy and Children

The shortest distance between two points is an intention.
—*John E. Upledger, DO, OMM*

The Twins

✿ The twins. That is the phrase that has appeared at least twice weekly in our schedule book for two years. We all know who they are even without their first names because of their unique circumstance. They were connected at the crowns of their heads in the rarest form of conjoinment, called craniopagus. These are the little boys whom the world came to know as "the Egyptian twins."

The World Craniofacial Foundation funded the boys' care and travel to Dallas, Texas, while a team of physicians, surgeons, and various specialists evaluated and discussed the possibility of separation surgery. Dr. Kenneth Salyer, a prominent craniofacial surgeon, referred the boys to us.

When we were asked if we would evaluate and treat them, we were thrilled for the opportunity. Since we are CranioSacral Therapists, the process promised to be even more intriguing. Since there was no blueprint to follow, we were learning to trust our hands with what we felt.

The first time we saw Ahmed and Mohammed Ibrahim, they were carried in the arms of their two devoted nurses who had been with them since birth. Their bodies draped over the nurses' extended arms like an awkward, oversized package. We placed the twins on one of our six-foot-long padded therapy swings so we could evaluate their cranial systems and response to movement. Their eyes were wide, and they were very quiet. Ahmed sucked on his two fingers, a gesture we would come to know meant that he was scared. The boys were just fifteen months old, an age when most children have already learned to walk. They had rarely been off their backs.

Ahmed was the larger of the two boys and quite passive. He was positioned so that he could gaze straight up to the ceiling. Developmentally he appeared to be around four months of age. He could move all of his extremities, although he appeared to prefer more passive social interaction. With even very slight swimming, his eyes flickered with rapid nystagmus fifty percent of the time, and he had very poor tolerance for movement. He had never played with his feet and was unable to hold his own bottle to eat. Functionally he appeared very weak, with little motivation to move.

Mohammed was the more active of the two boys, yet he also had very poor tolerance to movement. Nystagmus was present seventy-five percent of the time, and he demonstrated a strong right-sided neglect. He also had an entrapped vagus nerve and a very difficult time eating. He seemed to be surviving primarily from the food that his brother consumed.

Ahmed served as an efficient anchor for Mohammed. Despite Mohammed's attempts to roll onto his left side, he could not overpower his larger brother, who was perfectly content to lie still. When we placed both boys on their stomachs, Mohammed would push into extension, raising Ahmed's head with him. As the boys grew, there was more than one occasion when Ahmed inadvertently manipulated Mohammed's neck with a sudden roll.

The boys each had unique cranial systems. Their anatomy was such that they shared a sagittal sinus, and each had one jugular vein draining the blood from one into the other. Early CT scans suggested that they also shared a small portion of brain matter; by the time they had surgery, however, this did not appear to be the case. Their skulls and upper cervical vertebrae were twisted and flattened due to their unique positioning, and none of the suture lines were in the correct place.

Ahmed's cranial rhythm ran faster than his brother's, between eight and nine cycles per minute (cpm). He had greater flexion than extension, with a strong torsion to the right, from his sacrum all the way up into his cranial vault. His occipital base was flattened, and his head was quite wide.

Mohammed ran a little slower than Ahmed by about half a cpm (seven to eight times a minute), and he had more extension. A strong rotational force was present throughout both boys' bodies, similar to a towel being twisted. Initially there was minimal differentiation between their heads, where a cleft would later develop with the help of CranioSacral Therapy (CST).

When we first started working with the boys, we believed that we would either make a difference so that surgery could occur and have a greater chance of success, or we would be able to improve the quality of their lives so that they would at least be more mobile. We really didn't know what to expect. We just knew that we were going to give it our best shot and provide a lot of positive intention.

After the first treatment, the boys were smiling and moving more. Their nystagmus had decreased dramatically, and they could now tolerate swimming. Mohammed appeared to notice his right arm a little more, and both boys would reach up over their heads toward the other.

After six treatments, each had demonstrated a tremendous jump in his development. They looked more like eight-month-old boys, and both began playing with their hands and feet. They could get onto their tummies and push up into a crawling position. Even Ahmed was moving more and attempting to crawl. Mohammed had started to eat on his own and was beginning to gain weight.

Over the next several months, the surgeons decided that operating was a viable option, and they agreed to do it. By the time the boys went into separation surgery, they had been treated a minimum of two or three times a week with CST for more than a year. All treatments included a team of two to four therapists, all of whom had spent a week in Florida for an Intensive Program. Dr. John [Upledger] had also come to visit and treat the twins in Dallas.

The boys were ready. They were strong, happy, and healthy. They could stand up over a ball or swing and make walking movements. Even though they had to be in the hospital for several months while their skin was expanded to cover the incision sites, they remained infection-free and in good spirits. Whenever we came in to see them they would extend their arms to us with big smiles.

Two days after surgery we were able to get our hands on the boys, even though they would remain sedated and asleep for the next two weeks. Their rhythms were strong, and we knew they were going to be all right.

The operation had gone better than anyone had ever expected (except for us). There was minimal bleeding during the procedure; they were able to come out of sedation sooner than doctors had anticipated; and they progressed quickly. There were essentially no complications for the scope of the procedure, and their brains ended up being separate after all.

We continue to see the boys now as outpatients in our clinic. Mohammed is crawling well with minimal right-sided weakness and is walking with assistance. Both boys can sit independently and are talking up a storm—in three languages! Ahmed is starting to stand more. We are confident they will be walking by the time they go back to Egypt.

There is no question for us that the CranioSacral Therapy made a huge impact in these two boys' lives, as well as the lives of many others. In a world of territoriality, a diverse group of people came together to share their talents and time, bridging the gap between mainstream and complementary medicine in order to improve the quality of life for these twins. This is truly a time in which anything is possible with the right intention.

Suzanne Aderholt, OTR, CST
Dallas, Texas
CranioSacral Therapy Practitioner since 1997

Sally Fryer, PT, CST
Dallas, Texas
CranioSacral Therapy Practitioner since 1998

Ella

✿ *Sally Sederstrom:* We're certain that something greater than all of us brought Signy Erickson into our lives. She began treating our daughter Ella in early 2002, just before Ella turned two. Ella's now a happy, healthy, four-year-old who has, and will likely always have, significant physical and cognitive challenges. But there's no doubt in our hearts and minds that she would have much greater medical and emotional problems today if Signy had not been treating her.

When Ella began CranioSacral Therapy, we knew she had delays. But it wasn't until just before her third birthday that she was diagnosed with Rett syndrome (RS). The National Institute of Neurological Disorders and Stroke defines this as a "childhood neurodevelopmental disorder characterized by normal early development followed by loss of purposeful use of the hands, distinctive hand movements, slowed brain and head growth, gait abnormalities, seizures, and mental retardation." It is caused by a gene mutation that occurs before birth.

Ella's development has followed a pretty typical pattern for children with RS, although the specialists say she is "high-functioning Rett."

Walking became Ella's main mode of transportation just after she turned three. She doesn't speak, and isn't expected to, although she is very expressive. Most girls with RS have seizures and breathing disorders. Ella has neither, and we're convinced she doesn't because of CranioSacral Therapy.

As we look back at Ella's development, there were early signs of Rett syndrome. Typical of RS, Ella's motor and social development seemed to follow the usual schedule until she was about four months old. At nine months, she was only sitting, could not roll over, and seemed frightened to attempt any movement outside of where she could reach with her hands. Between her six- and nine-month well-child checkups, her head circumference did not grow.

When Ella was eleven months old, we began weekly physical and occupational therapy. This one-on-one work was helpful. After about six months, she began her version of a crawl, a sort of bunny hop. She progressed physically, but was frustrated and seemed to be in her own world. She was apathetic to toys and wouldn't interact with her sisters. It was often hard to calm crying spells, and she didn't want to cuddle. She had some autistic-like behaviors, such as rocking back and forth and side to side, and banging her head on the floor or on someone's head. She did have great eye contact, and everyone we asked about autism said she was "too social."

When we started to ask what else we could do, a variety of people mentioned CranioSacral Therapy. The physical therapist at Ella's Early Intervention program referred us to Signy Erickson.

We took a very frustrated and sad child to Signy, yet Ella was immediately comfortable with her. She sat calmly on Signy's lap at the first session while Signy and I talked. I couldn't tell Signy was doing anything, but I remember her saying, "Oh, that was a good release." Ella left calm and happy, and I was eager for her next visit.

Signy Erickson: When Ella was carried in, the first thing I noticed was that she seemed fairly disinterested in her surroundings, although she did look me in the eye to check me out. The main thing I worked with in that first visit was her cranium, which had a very unbalanced craniosacral rhythm and a strong restriction at the coronal suture.

At Ella's second visit, she showed much more curiosity about me and about things in the room. Sally mentioned that Ella seemed more in tune and alert, and her head banging had decreased. I felt an incredible connection with Ella, and still do, but find it impossible to adequately put into words. It felt like she knew that I was there to help her, and was grateful for it. It also seemed like we somehow knew each other on another level.

Within six weeks of starting treatment, Ella pulled herself up to a standing position by herself for the first time. She started to show much more interest in moving, in investigating her surroundings, and in holding longer eye contact. Most of all, Ella was beginning to be known for her giggling. She also was sleeping better. For a few visits she would start to cry when it was time to leave the office. We finally realized it was because she didn't want to leave!

Sally: Signy has now treated Ella for almost two and a half years, and we are convinced that without it, Ella would be far more affected by Rett syndrome.

After six months of CranioSacral Therapy, Ella's head circumference grew almost two centimeters, and has continued to grow. Ella's EEG does show atypical brain patterns, but she does not take antiseizure drugs and has never had a seizure. (Most children with RS have seizures and are on medication.)

We're also convinced that Signy has helped Ella develop emotionally. These two have a bond that goes far beyond CranioSacral Therapy. Ella walks into the treatment room an extremely happy child, greets Signy with a hug, and offers a kiss and wave good-bye. She likes to cuddle and follow her sisters in their antics.

Ella has become very expressive and loves people, animals, and her surroundings. While unpurposeful hand movements, often hand-wringing, are characteristic of Rett syndrome, Ella claps instead, which is certainly a happy gesture.

Signy: It seems to those who know Ella that she has been "unlocked" both physically and emotionally. She still receives CranioSacral Therapy every three weeks or so. She continues to make strides in her motor skills and is starting to try to speak a few words. The frustrated child who was carried into the office for her first visit now walks in by herself, has a smile and huge twinkles in her eyes, and seems delighted to share her giggles with everyone. She brings a joy to us all.

Story by Sally Sederstrom and Signy Erickson
Submitted by Signy Erickson, DC, CST-D
Bend, Oregon
CranioSacral Therapy Practitioner since 1989

Persevering Through the Darkness

✿ It has been nine years since my son David attended the one-week Learning-Disabled Intensive Program at the innovative Upledger Institute Healthplex Clinical Services in Palm Beach Gardens, Florida.

At the start of the program, David's vocabulary was limited to various forms of "Da." By the end of the week, he was speaking three- to five-word sentences that were clearly audible, and he was beaming with newfound confidence and self-esteem.

Before my very eyes, by the hands of many compassionate and highly skilled therapists, our family's life was impacted beyond my greatest dreams and hopes.

Joyous expression now replaced the growing frustration and anger that had built up during David's first three years of life. Parental frustration, despair, and heartbreak started to melt away with a glimmer of hope that significant change would be long-lasting.

Meeting with Dr. John [Upledger] after this most intense, exhaustive, and exhilarating week of my life, I asked him, "What's next? Where do we go from here?"

Throughout the year and a half preceding this experience, we had played the rebound game with local osteopaths. They had done good work but never seemed to get to the core of the deep-seated pattern/dysfunction that prevented David's verbal expression. During this time I had seen David make slight minor improvements only to quickly regress to the original dysfunctional pattern. Deep inside me was that nagging fear that this would be no exception. Little did I know that this time there would be no regression!

Dr. John said with determined courage and optimism, "Go home and let David learn to talk in his own way and on his own terms." Could it be that simple and easy, I wondered?

I was torn inside. Ongoing speech therapy seemed obligatory. I remember the speech therapist saying, "How can he learn to talk if no one teaches him how?" She implied that I was being irresponsible, and guilt was directed my way for not acting in David's best interest.

When we got home from the clinic I followed Dr. John's recipe. David and I made up our own sounds, sang together, and repeated the names of the many things we explored. Day by day, he increased his ability to generate sounds of all types: a dog barking, a cat meowing, the hiss of the wind blowing, and new words of one and two syllables.

I continued to apply and use CranioSacral Therapy (CST) techniques and all forms of loving touch therapy that David would allow. I remember asking his permission to lay my healing hands on him. He said, "Yes, but just for five minutes." Well, to David that meant counting slowly to five and then saying, "We're done!"

At first I protested and felt frustrated. Then I remembered that CST is about *not* having an agenda. As a result, I have developed the best five- to ten-second CST treatment protocol that has ever been done! I have come to realize that miracles and effective treatments can come in very small timeframes. After all, it really is all about healing intention.

As David got older, I asked him what he remembered about this therapeutic experience when he was three years old. He recalled thinking that people were trying to hurt him during the initial stages of therapy. I can understand that. I can remember holding his squirming body to the table and telling him we were there for him and that we loved him—all this while three to five other therapists applied therapeutic techniques to his mind, body, and soul. I can imagine that it must have been distressing, threatening, and scary for a little boy of three to be on a massage table receiving treatments that were beyond his analytical understanding.

I am grateful for whatever it was that allowed our love and caring to penetrate David's resistance. Growth and recovery often involve pain and discomfort. When one can persevere through the darkness and terror, the light on the other side can bring great rewards and joy. Unconditional faith and trust is a wonderful thing.

At age four, David entered preschool. He received stimulation from a lot more kids his age, and his growth continued to expand. Before we knew it, songs were being sung in kindergarten, and the nightmares and dysfunctional patterns of David's first three years were quickly fading into oblivion.

David is now twelve years old. I often get asked how he is doing these days. He continues to be a straight-A student. He has been in choirs since grade school and has near-perfect pitch. He excels in all sports; soccer is his favorite. He empowers others on and off the field in ways I find difficult to put into words. David has lifelong friends and is continually making new friends. David is an inspiration to all who know him—especially to me.

When I see what David has gone through and the type of young adult he is becoming, it gives me faith and trust that the impossible can become possible. Thank you, Dr. John. Rest assured that as long as David and I continue to grow and thrive, your work and passion for growth, healing, and going where others have stopped will certainly go on. With healing hands and an open heart, let's all reach out and make this world a better place to live.

Phillip Henderson, CMT
Santa Rosa, California
CranioSacral Therapy Practitioner since 1991

CranioSacral and the Nervous Tic

Kay Suddeth, a friend of mine, called me one afternoon in November 2003 concerned about her daughter Mallory, who had developed a nervous head tic. This was not new to Kay. Mallory had had this same nervous tic as a child.

When Mallory was six years old, Kay noticed that she would shake her head quite often, as if she were playing with her ponytail. She soon realized that Mallory was not doing this on purpose. She had developed a nervous head tic that would come every four seconds. With this came some facial tics and excessive blinking. Kay was concerned; however, she felt there might be a correlation between the tics and her recent separation from her husband.

Mallory's oldest sister, Dominique, was the only one who could handle Mallory when she had a very bad episode. She would cradle her sister's head and put cold compresses on her with great love and devotion.

Kay had taken Mallory to different physicians but did not care for the Western medicine techniques. She felt that if the body were given enough time it might correct itself. She also felt that a more natural approach would be better. Kay was right. It took two years, but Mallory did outgrow the problem.

This time was different, though. Mallory was eighteen and pregnant. They were not sure why the nervous tics had returned, but they were so severe that Kay called a neurologist. It was going to take too long to get an appointment. About the same time, Mallory had seen her chiropractor for an adjustment. When Kay expressed her concerns to him, he recommended CranioSacral Therapy.

Kay knew that I had studied a variety of modalities, including CranioSacral Therapy, and so she called me. I agreed to see Mallory the next afternoon.

During the first session with her, I saw firsthand the severity of the nervous tics. Several times her head came out of my hands. After a few moments, the tics quieted down. There were several jerking motions throughout the body during that first session. Even with the different jerking and twitching, Mallory fell asleep for a short period of time. The first session lasted almost two hours.

Mallory let me know later that the length and frequency of the tics had slowed down at a remarkable pace. By the third session her tics were almost completely gone. "It really works!" Mallory said. "I feel so much better. I still have a few tics every once and a while, but they are so infrequent that I don't notice them."

"We are delighted with the results," Kay said.

I continued to work on Mallory once a month until about six weeks before the baby came. During delivery, the nervous tics returned with some severity. Afterward, Mallory saw a therapist closer to her home and continues to receive CranioSacral Therapy as needed.

Mary Glesige, LMT
Nashville, Tennessee
CranioSacral Therapy Practitioner since 2003

From Frustration to Function

Being a parent of an ADD (attention deficit disorder) child has many special challenges. To tell the child to get up and get ready for school is nearly impossible at times. Simple steps must be given: "It's time to get up. First, put on your clothes. Next, come to eat. Now, brush your teeth."

Processing complex commands seems so easy if your brain allows you to do this. But when you realize that your child is just not capable of this, it breaks your heart. And unless you realize that your child has special needs, you and your family are subject to many frustrating and emotional moments.

I am that mother, but I am also a physical therapist who took CranioSacral Therapy in 1993. It was in that class where I heard that the temporal bones may play a part in ADD and learning disabilities. My son Gabe, in addition to the ADD, had degrees of visual-perceptual difficulties, dyslexia, and dyscalculia.

Armed only with this training from the beginning class, I volunteered my son to be my guinea pig. Luckily, my son fell promptly asleep when I got to the frontal lift, which allowed me to listen to the cranial bone better. Neither of his temporal bones was moving well, and the right side was very immobile. I worked for about an hour and a half on my son that night and was able to get motion in all of his cranial bones, especially freeing up temporal motion. My husband carried my deeply sleeping son off to bed.

The next morning, before I could launch my routine of simple, single-step commands to start our day, my son was up and fully ready for the school day. Not once did I have to remind him what to do next. To our great surprise, his self-organization continued. He would wake up on his own and get ready without asking. I also noticed that homework hassles were becoming nonexistent.

Of all these things, the most remarkable moment for me came some years later, when Gabe was fifteen. He said that he remembered the day after I first worked on him, because the pressure in his head had vanished and he could think better.

CranioSacral Therapy was the key that unlocked Gabe's frustrating world of not remembering what comes next and always trying to hide the fact that you don't remember what your teachers just told you to do.

My son is now nineteen and serves as an Honor Guard to a Four-Star United States General in the U.S. Army. He continues to be on time and organized.

I have continued my quest to learn more about CranioSacral Therapy because of my son and my other children. If we can help just one child and parent, it is such a gift.

Chloe Sluis, PT
Auburn, California
CranioSacral Therapy Practitioner since 1993

Changing Lives, One at a Time

✿ CranioSacral Therapy has been a life-changing experience for me, as well as those I've treated over the years. So many people have been positively affected by this work, and I am so grateful to be a part of their lives in this way.

A young boy named Robbie* comes to mind. He was about two and a half years old when I first began to treat him. He had been diagnosed with autism and also suffered from chronic ear infections and respiratory problems. His birth had been normal. He received occupational and speech therapies at preschool.

At his first treatment, Robbie gave his mother and me a screaming session that let us know quite clearly that he didn't want to be in my office. His mother was holding him on her lap while she sat on my massage table.

With my hands on Robbie's thoracic diaphragm, I listened. There were restrictions in his lungs, which was a little unbelievable given how well they had just worked. His head felt like a rock; nothing was moving very much, not membranes or cranial bones. It felt as though he had been living with one giant headache.

The screaming was ear-piercing. We could tolerate about twenty minutes before I closed the session with diaphragm releases and still points.

The next week Robbie was back. The scenario was similar, yet the screaming didn't last quite as long, and he tolerated a bit more hands-on treatment. With his mother holding him, I treated what I could reach. This time he allowed me to begin working on his head after a few diaphragm releases and still points. They stayed about forty minutes that time.

Robbie returned weekly for more therapy. He continued to tolerate more and more hands-on time. His cranial vault began to

---

*Name changed to protect client confidentiality

loosen up and maintain some of the new releases. The screaming stopped, and he began to tolerate more treatment with little scheduled breaks. We negotiated positioning. Though he continued to need his mother's touch, he was now satisfied by her sitting next to the table, holding his hand.

As time went on, Robbie began to feel the difference in his body. He no longer needed his mother to continually touch him, and she reported differences in his behavior at home. Robbie seemed to quiet more easily and was more attentive and cooperative.

The therapist at Robbie's school began to report that he was more verbal, not just vocal; his eye-tracking skills were improved; he had a greater frustration tolerance; and he was beginning to tolerate interaction with other children in more positive ways.

As the months passed, Robbie's progress continued. In preparation for his appointments, his mother would tell him that he was coming to see me. She said he would respond by putting his hands on his head and saying, "Shyamala." When he got to my office, he would run in, jump up on the table unassisted, and lie supine the entire hour. His mother would not even have to be in the room with him. She got to sit in the waiting room and have an hour to herself to read and relax. Robbie's body had learned that he could feel better and have better coping mechanisms when he got consistent treatment.

I treated Robbie for just over a year before he moved away, yet I think of him often. I feel very blessed, reveling in the fact that such profound, productive changes can happen in one person's life. It truly is an honor to be a part of someone's life in that way.

Shyamala Strack, OTR/L, CST-D
Atlanta, Georgia
CranioSacral Therapy Practitioner since 1991

The Miracle of Morgann:
A Story of Love and CST

Morgann was born February 19, 2002, with a number of problems. Due to a complication during amniocentesis, a significant volume of amniotic fluid had been lost while she was *in utero.* As a result, Morgann was unable to extend her limbs or turn around in the womb. She essentially took on the shape of the inner womb outline. Her neck was hyperextended backward; her spine was in the shape of a large C; her limbs had no range of motion; her chest had not expanded enough to breath normally; and her swallow reflex was impaired.

At the time of birth, Morgann's APGAR score was one. (A normal score is five.) She was intubated and sent to the Neonatal Intensive Care Unit (NICU). The prognosis was extremely poor.

Still in NICU four months later, Morgann was faring poorly. She required constant care that included a tracheotomy, mechanical ventilator, gastrostomy, and feeding tube insertion. Hypersensitive to external sights and sounds, she would "crash" (experience almost immediate respiratory and cardiac distress) with any stimulation. She was not expected to ever breathe or swallow on her own, nor was she expected to respond or develop mentally or physically.

No one provided genuine encouragement, and on several occasions Mom and Dad were actively discouraged from bonding with this very fragile newborn. Ignoring suggestions, Morgann's parents continued to visit their new daughter daily.

Those in charge of her care (doctors and the insurance company) advised the parents to place Morgann in an institution for the severely brain-damaged. Reluctantly Mom and Dad visited the recommended institution. Afterward they decided that if their beloved child were to die, it would be at home with her family and not in a sterile institution.

At this point, Mom and Dad turned to Just 4 Kids, a local pediatric home-care agency with which I work part-time. When I met Morgann for the first time, she had been home from the hospital four days. Although she was indeed in distress, she had already lived twice the expected forty-eight hours.

After I worked with Morgann through several night shifts, I requested and was given her parents' permission to administer CranioSacral Therapy. Dad's assistance was enlisted to hold Morgann's abdomen upright while I worked in the cranial base area. The extreme C shape of her spine meant that Morgann had been unable to lie on her back since birth. By the second session, Morgann slept deeply throughout each treatment.

I applied CST techniques of the basic 10-Step Protocol, direction of energy, V-spread, etc. Specific attention was initially directed to the back, neck, and cranial base. Dramatic results could be felt very rapidly and could be seen after about ten treatments, when she was able to lie on her flat back.

There clearly existed an impaction of the occiput onto the vertebrae. As the CranioSacral Therapist, I experienced awe when the cranial base finally released gently and completely. To see this infant sound asleep and flat on her back for the first time was truly a source of joy, achieved with gentle touch and energy.

Her primary pediatrician considered Morgann a possible "failure to thrive" infant because she had gained only minimal weight for the first nine months of her life. This suddenly changed, however, and she began to grow and even thrive over the next month. In fact, the pediatrician thought that she was gaining too rapidly and put her on a diet!

The prediction by the pulmonologist that Morgann would never breathe without the ventilator was soon proven incorrect as well. Five months and five days after leaving NICU, she spontaneously reached up one evening and removed the ventilator tubing from her trach. (She had been receiving twice-weekly CST sessions at this point.) Dad and I watched her body, her pulse rate, and her oxygen saturation for signs of respiratory distress. I explained to Dad that in a few minutes Morgann would show some indication of intolerance to being off the ventilator; at that time we would reconnect the machine. She breathed normally until slight fatigue seemed to begin—after thirty-seven minutes off the ventilator. Morgann's ventilator was completely discontinued some months later. Even the pulmonologist was impressed!

Intellectually, Morgann has progressed extremely well. Her recognition of toys and people, her ability to intercept and push away a fine-gauge suction catheter approaching her tracheostomy, her ability to focus on words on a book page, her smile when she's happy—all indicate a mental development greater than her chronological age.

At twenty-two months of age, it is apparent that Morgann's limbs will be shorter than normal, and her physical developmental landmarks are delayed. The people who care for her on a daily basis believe her landmark delays are secondary to that physically slow growth start.

Morgann had also been diagnosed with severe hearing impairment. In the last eighteen months, there has been significant change. She now startles with loud noises and turns toward the sound of her daddy's voice when he speaks in another room. The power on her hearing aids has been reduced twice so far.

Morgann remains off the ventilator and needs only a very small oxygen support. She receives speech and physical therapies. Her hip and shoulder range of motion has been one hundred percent since she was six months old. And she still receives CST at least twice per month.

This child amazes all who come in contact with her. She continues to defy all negative prognosis statements by her doctors. A decorative banner at the top of the wall nearest her crib states in large letters: "With God all things are possible."

My life and my world have grown immeasurably since I began studying CranioSacral Therapy. I thank Dr. Upledger and the staff of The Upledger Institute for making both my world and Morgann's a better, more joyous place for so many people.

Jean Reid, RNC, LMT
West Palm Beach, Florida
CranioSacral Therapy Practitioner since 2000

Restored Symmetry Refutes Diagnosis

As a physical therapist working with developmentally disabled students, one of my more enjoyable responsibilities is screening infants and toddlers to determine if they need therapy services. One infant I particularly recall was five-month-old Ronan.

Ronan was brought to the school by his mother and an early intervention (EI) specialist, a teacher who follows children diagnosed at birth with potential developmental problems. He had a medical diagnosis of congenital torticollis. As soon as I looked at Ronan I noticed that his head was misshapen, with flatness on the right parietal bone. Also, his frontal bone seemed to be more prominent on the right. During my physical therapy evaluation I could not find any signs typical of torticollis, such as sternocleidomastoid muscle tightness or a side-bent and rotated head position. He appeared to be developing normally for his age.

Typically in such a situation I would give the mother encouragement that everything appeared normal and send them on their way with a written summary for the referring physician. However, I could not ignore the asymmetry in Ronan's head. Cautiously I asked Mom if she had noticed it. She said that she had first noted it at birth and was told Ronan would outgrow it. She further stated that she did not think he was outgrowing it after five months.

Asking about the birth process, I discovered that Ronan had had a hard time exiting the birth canal. Again with caution, I suggested to both the EI specialist and Mom that he might benefit from a form of therapy that uses very light touch to help the body correct itself.

At this point the EI specialist said, "Oh, you mean CranioSacral Therapy! I was able to watch another client receive a treatment and it was amazing." Mom had also heard of CranioSacral Therapy (CST) but didn't know much about it. I gave her a short description of it, and she was very receptive to the idea. Ronan also seemed receptive. When I first touched his head he immediately went into a still point.

My problem now was whom to refer them to. In my position I was only allowed to refer out the early intervention cases, not to treat them. I wrote my evaluation summary and recommended that Ronan be seen by a therapist who was trained to treat children using CST to address the asymmetry in his head. Both Mom and the specialist seemed to think this would be a good option.

A few days later, the EI specialist called me and stated that the pediatrician did not agree with my assessment and that Ronan was to see a torticollis specialist. He would be fitted with a special helmet to reshape his head. She relayed that Mom was very upset and really wanted to try CST. She asked me if I could see him privately. I told her I would think about it. I had not yet taken the pediatric CST course, but I had all the prerequisites and used it regularly on the school-aged students.

After about thirty minutes I realized that I was meant to work with this child. One, he lived five minutes from my home. Two, his mom did not want to use a helmet. And three, they were asking for my help. I told them that I would see Ronan in his home at no charge and see what happened.

Our first visit was a few days later. Mom took "before" pictures. She told me that he had an appointment with the specialist in one month. During that first visit Ronan was very actively practicing his newly acquired motor skill of rolling. I managed to detect tightness in his sacrum, cranial base, and left coronal and squamous sutures. I did my best to distract, hold, and follow this moving target for about twenty minutes. Mom and I decided that we would try once-weekly visits for the remaining three weeks until the specialist appointment.

The second visit was the turning point. Ronan seemed determined to show off his rolling skills again until I held his occiput and sacrum. He suddenly stopped moving and went into a still point. I followed a very wonderful unwinding that lasted for about five minutes. During this time he smiled and lay very still. Then, just as suddenly, he resumed his calisthenics. Ronan was telling me that treatment was done for the day.

When I returned a week later, Mom said she thought his head shape was rounding out a bit. Indeed, the right parietal bone appeared more rounded. I also noticed that the restriction to the left parietal lift was much less than it was initially.

On the fourth and last visit before the specialist appointment, I could not feel a restriction to either the parietal or frontal lift. In fact, I really had a hard time finding much to treat. Ronan's mom took "after" pictures, and I asked her to call to let me know how the appointment went.

The specialist apparently looked at the pictures and agreed that the cranial asymmetry was not significant. A helmet was not pre-scribed. I offered to continue to see Ronan if Mom would like me to, but she declined.

I am so glad that I listened to my intuition and went ahead and treated Ronan. It was as if he was telling me during that first screening what to do when he went into a still point. Even the fact that he ended up being screened by someone who knew that CST could help his condition seems more than a coincidence.

Pat Churavy, PT
Avon, Ohio
CranioSacral Therapy Practitioner since 1999

No More Earaches

From the day my daughter Jessica was born she had constant ear infections. We'd go to the pediatrician, who would give us a round of amoxicillin, which then progressed to Zithromax, which ultimately led to her *always* being on some form of antibiotic. This went on for the first three years of her life, even prompting a myringotomy with ear tubes, much to my consternation, shortly after her second birthday. That lasted for about three months, until the tubes fell out and it started all over again.

Shortly after her third birthday, I was in Dallas taking three Myofascial Release classes over a period of ten days. On the third day of classes, the instructors started talking about CranioSacral Therapy (CST). They demonstrated the 10-Step Protocol, which we then practiced for the next couple of hours and once again the following day. They mentioned that CST is very helpful in alleviating ear infections.

The Friday before I was to come home, my wife called to say that she had taken Jessica to an ear-nose-throat (ENT) specialist who told her that Jessica had a complete bilateral blockage. She then proceeded to tell me that they had scheduled a second operation for ear tubes in ten days.

When I got home, I could tell that Jessica had been crying from the pain and was running a fever. That night and for the next five days, for approximately twenty minutes a day, I attempted to employ the rudimentary CST techniques we had been taught. I didn't know if they would help, but I knew that I didn't want my daughter to have to repeat the hellish trauma she had been subjected to barely a year before.

The next Tuesday, we went back to the ENT for a pre-op examination. He looked first in one ear and then the other with his scope. His only comment was, "Hmm." Then he did a tympanogram on both ears and asked, "What was the matter with her?" We told him that she had a complete bilateral blockage of both ears. To this he questioningly remarked, "Really?" He then put Jessica in the audio booth and ran a full audiogram on her. At the conclusion he said, "Her hearing is perfect. There's nothing wrong." Then he said something that I'm sure pained him very much to say: "I'm canceling her surgery."

The doctor asked me what we had done to Jessica, and I replied that I had done CranioSacral Therapy on her. He said he had never seen such a rapid recovery from such a severe infection. He commented that he'd heard of CranioSacral Therapy being used for autism, but never for ear infections. I offered him my card and told him I'd appreciate any referrals he could send my way. Needless to say, I never heard from him, and we haven't seen him since. That was seven years ago, and Jessica has never had another ear infection!

Within the next couple of weeks, I scheduled my first formal CranioSacral Therapy class through The Upledger Institute and haven't looked back since. Learning of CST was the best thing that ever happened to my bodyworking career and certainly for my daughter. I have since worked on my nephew for the same reason, with exactly the same results. My stepsister was ecstatic. CST has a faithful following in our family. Thank you, Dr. John!

Chuck Olson, RMT
Bellville, Texas
CranioSacral Therapy Practitioner since 1998

CST Unlocks Response Mechanism

✿ After a totally normal development, my seventeen-month-old daughter Kasey lost the ability to speak, comprehend language, or make eye contact. She also began making strange sounds and gestures.

I started taking her to a physical therapist named Kris for Cranio-Sacral Therapy (CST) when she was three years old, basically because I was desperate. This was back in 1996, when I had to travel nearly four hours each way and pay almost entirely out of my own pocket.

After more than twenty hours of therapy, I was thinking that our next visit to Kris might be our last if I didn't see any results. The truth is, I probably would have quit sooner, but I kept feeling like something very special was going on. Plus, being surrounded by CST and those therapists just felt right.

On the day of decision, Kris was working on Kasey when I heard, "Oh my, the top of her cranium just shifted and is now sitting on the bottom where it belongs!" I smiled politely and told myself that these people were all insane and that I would not be back.

The next morning, just to humor myself, I decided to check out Kasey's head, which had been clearly lopsided. When I made pigtails, I always had to move the part to one side of her head in order to make the two sides look even. When I went to make the pigtails that morning, though, I couldn't believe what I saw. Her head was totally normal! I started to scream and immediately got on the phone to Kris. "You did it!" I screamed. "You fixed her head!" Kris was a little confused and said, "Yes, I know. I thought I told you that yesterday."

At that point, there were no functional changes, just structural. I can only imagine the impact of that strain on Kasey's brain, blood vessels, and intracranial membranes.

A few months later, when Kasey was four, we saw another PT

named Chris, who told me he was going to "unlock Kasey's sphenoid bone and free up her pituitary gland." By this point in time I trusted these therapists totally.

Sure enough, the next morning Kasey demonstrated the ability to respond to language, a skill she had never had before. I was always told that I should speak to her as if she understood me, even though I would feel like I was talking to the wall. Well, that morning, Kasey followed through with the appropriate action when I reminded her that she needed to wipe after using the toilet. I was shocked! I continued testing her. First I asked her to turn off the light, which she did. I then went around the house making various requests, all of which Kasey did exactly as I told her.

This work is absolutely amazing! I began to realize that Kasey did understand me the whole time, but, prior to treatment, she was unable to get her body to follow my commands.

Another wonderful thing occurred at age five. Kasey's top teeth were not visible when she smiled; they were hidden behind her top lip. One day while working with her, another therapist named Sharon said that the maxilla was tilted upward. She did her thing, and within two days Kasey's top teeth began to descend; within a week they were totally visible! A beautiful smile!

Needless to say, CranioSacral Therapy has given me many beautiful smiles.

Eileen Rahamim, LAC
Staten Island, New York
CranioSacral Therapy Practitioner since 1999

Miracle After a Mauling

✿ Returning home from a class on Clinical Applications of CranioSacral Therapy (CST) for Pediatrics, I was put to task. A woman named Melinda★ came into the clinic to purchase a bottle of herbs for her friend. Her son Toby★ was with her. As he walked across the room I saw that he was severely twisted in the low back, pelvis, and hips, resulting in a limp, no heel strike, and a labored gait. He was also quite withdrawn, difficult to talk to, tense, distant, angry, and wanted nothing in his space.

I inquired about the condition of the child. Melinda informed me that Toby had been mauled by a horse about three months prior. He had experienced a traumatic event of violent twisting, shaking, flailing, and tossing. The horse had bitten out part of the vastus medialis muscle just inferior to the sartorius (inner leg above the knee). The injuries sustained had resulted in loss of muscle mass and skin. At first look, the doctors thought he would lose his leg.

Toby's next step was Botox shots, physical therapy, and then three surgeries, along with a lot of psychological appointments. Melinda did not want to take this invasive path; she wanted another option. I shared with her the possible benefits of CST for Toby. Melinda understood there might be criticism from the doctors but elected to give CST a try.

The first time I treated Toby, he was concerned about the therapy hurting. We talked and played. I showed him the disarticulating skull along with three sizes of sand-filled, shiny, stuffed lizards and two frog toys he could play with. He was passive in movement and had a lot of questions.

During the session, his little body worked very hard. He felt many "weird" sensations as each release occurred. He had a look of profound inner change following that short session. He was calm

---

★Names changed to protect patient confidentiality

and moved with more ease. His mother called the following day stating that Toby had slept through the entire night with no episodes of night terrors.

The physical therapist working with Toby was instrumental in allowing Melinda a chance to try out CST on Toby. The PT had heard of The Upledger Institute and of my work, so she took the second seat, measuring Toby's progress and working to regain his coordination and strength. One of the more stunning measurements, I am told, was a ten-degree improvement of the range of motion in Toby's ankle in one session of CST. He could now strike his heel.

The other astounding progress I observed was in emotional changes. Toby went from killing the toy lizards, tearing apart the skulls, and throwing the pieces all over the room, to racing with the clock to put the skulls together and having all the lizards and frogs work together. He went from pushing me out of his space to hugging and giving me notes with "I love you" written on them. He also raised his grades to A's and set an example in his class. In less than six months from this mauling and less than three months of receiving CST, Toby was playing basketball.

Today, Toby's little body is aligned and full of life. He has a scar medially above the knee, but that is a small disfigurement to deal with. All of this dramatic improvement occurred in about three months of weekly sessions.

Toby and his family moved away the following summer. His mother, who stays in touch, told me that Toby (now eight) is playing football this year. He is calm, active, gets straight A's, and the leg that was injured is growing faster than the other one. The only concern is with the skin graft and a growing body, but so far the leg is accommodating the growth with no problems.

Before he moved away Toby gave me a key chain with a little sand-filled lizard on the other end. It was about the size of the small one he had identified with throughout his sessions. As he gave it to me, tears welled in his eyes, he swallowed hard, and he gave me a big hug. I know this experience will be a very special part of this child's life forever. As for me, it strengthens my stand on healing, the miracle of life, and the great Hippocratic oath: Do no harm.

Beth Jezik, RMT
Killeen, Texas
CranioSacral Therapy Practitioner since 1995

And the Cocoon Hatched

❀ Joe is a ten-year-old boy who emerged about five months ago from the "cocoon" he was living in.

He lived close by in my neighborhood, yet I had very seldom seen him play outside. One night, a group of us were together, celebrating a neighborhood couple's wedding anniversary. Some of them knew I was a massage therapist. I began explaining that I also do Reiki, CranioSacral Therapy, and Lymph Drainage Therapy. All of a sudden my neighbors were very intrigued, and I was placed under a spotlight.

This was my opportunity to educate my neighbors on regaining balance and wellness through these wonderful, complementary, natural alternatives. Most of them had no idea that these therapies went much further than just relaxation purposes. Their understanding of bodywork went from trivially curious to profoundly edifying. I noticed that Marilyn was the most attentive.

A couple of weeks later, she came to me with her silent, remote son, Joe. Her eyes told me that she didn't know what else to do. Her voice told me that Joe was dealing with ADHD (attention deficit hyperactivity disorder) and Aderal side effects. He had problems sleeping and eating. Most upsetting to them, however, were his increasingly frequent migraine headaches.

Marilyn told me that her son was usually very active, but during the onset of a migraine headache he would curl inward, like he was in a cocoon, and go to a corner and cry. There he would keep himself isolated from everyone and everything. She would immediately get ice and pills for her aching son. This didn't just happen at home, either. The problem was disabling him in school, in his relationships with friends, and in his favorite sport, basketball.

It took only one twenty-minute CranioSacral Therapy (CST)

---

*Name changed to protect client confidentiality

session to get raving reviews from Mom. That afternoon, Joe went straight for dinner, fell asleep before bedtime, and slept the whole night without interruption. Kids are wonderful!

Regaining balance is so much easier when conditions haven't had enough time to settle in and make it more difficult to liberate your mind and body from crystallizing dysfunction.

Four days later, Joe had a follow-up CST session. The same boy who first came in looking down at the floor gave me a hug and didn't lose eye contact. He was most cooperative and relaxed on the table. Evaluation showed that his sphenoid was almost balanced. (It was all over the place the first time we met.) His cranial base needed more work as a preventive measure for headaches. I just did three more fine-tunings, but the migraine headaches never came back after that first CranioSacral Therapy session.

Joe's loving mother, Marilyn, recently said to me, "He's so happy. It's like he broke out of a cocoon and is now free."

Vanessa Martin, MT
Bayamon, Puerto Rico
CranioSacral Therapy Practitioner since 2001

The Case of the Disappearing Scoliosis

✿ Katy's appointment for CranioSacral Therapy was a desperate last stop before undergoing surgery for severe juvenile-onset scoliosis.

At age fourteen, her life had changed dramatically. Once a very active and athletic young lady, she'd given up both gymnastics and soccer over the past year. Her painful back muscles would no longer allow for agile movement. More recently, severe headaches were affecting her schoolwork. Once a top student, she could no longer visually focus or concentrate for any length of time because her head always hurt.

Katy's pediatric orthopedist had given up on the noninvasive options. He'd had her in a back brace and physical therapy, but nothing seemed to slow down her increasing scoliotic curve. He told Katy and her parents that surgery was the only answer.

The plan was to fuse vertebrae. According to the doctor, the result would be less pain, though it was unlikely that the young girl would be able to return to her former sports—certainly not gymnastics.

Arriving at my office, Katy's mom seemed rushed and distracted. She and Katy's father were going through a divorce. Her plan was to have her soon-to-be ex-husband pick up their daughter after the appointment so that he'd be forced to pay for the treatment. Mom dashed out the door, and Katy was left with me, a total stranger, hoping to help her.

Amazingly, this girl, who seemed so small and fragile, lay down on my table and appeared incredibly serene. I was impressed. Her faith in this process, of which she knew next to nothing, was palpable.

Looking back, all I recall doing was supporting her spine in a dural tube hold, one hand under her sacrum, the other under her head. I may have moved my hands slightly during the session, perhaps a bit more toward her mid-back. Mostly I just sat still and held her. Time passed, and Katy's entire back began to feel like melting wax. It warmed and liquefied, and suddenly I felt like my hands were floating in water. Katy opened her eyes and said quietly, "Wow, something weird is happening."

One week later, Katy arrived at my office with news. "I feel completely different," she told me. Her headaches were gone and her energy had returned. Out of curiosity, I asked her if she would mind bending forward slightly so that I could assess the curvature of her spine. It was completely straight! I was amazed. I checked again. Still straight.

We did the second session as planned, but nothing dramatic happened, and that was fine. We both agreed it felt like a confirmation of the changes her body had achieved the week before. After the session, Katy and I went eagerly out to the waiting room to report to her dad that her spine looked and felt straight. Her father looked doubtful. He paid me and said he'd let her mother know.

The following day I spoke to Katy's mother by phone; she sounded tired and almost disinterested. She told me that Katy would be going back to the orthopedist soon; he would decide what to do. Weeks went by and I heard nothing.

Finally, the call came from Katy's mom. She was ecstatic! The doctor had taken X-rays of Katy's spine and was dumbfounded. He told them that if he didn't know absolutely that the X-rays were from the same girl, he never would have believed it. Her spine was normal.

Needless to say, the surgery was canceled. I saw Katy about once a year after that, until she went away to college. When we last spoke, she told me that a chiropractic adjustment every so often was all she needed to stay healthy and pain-free.

I never heard from her orthopedist.

Margery Chessare, LMT
Greenfield Center, New York
CranioSacral Therapy Practitioner since 1995

Baby Ella Finds What She Needs

❀ *Susan Hartung:* My beautiful daughter, Ella, was born full-term and seemingly healthy in April 2002. The day following her birth, however, she was diagnosed with a heart defect after her pediatrician found a significant murmur.

Tetralogy of Fallot (TOF) is a malformation of the heart consisting of four components: a narrowing of the pulmonary valve, a large hole between the ventricles, a dilated aorta, and a thickening of the right ventricle. Ella's heart was repaired successfully when she was almost three months old. Following the surgery, she spent eight days in the hospital. This may not seem like a long time, but for a newborn in early development it can cause quite a setback.

To get Ella "back on her feet," I sought assistance right away from an early intervention program in my county for children born with disabilities. After working with Ella for several months, the occupational therapist recommended CranioSacral Therapy (CST). I did some initial research on the Internet. I was not at all familiar with CST but am always open to alternative healing forms. In talking to other people about it, Sandy Prantl's name was mentioned several times as the one to see. I took that as a sign.

Because of Ella's surgery, I was not able to give her "tummy time." She was always on her back and would rarely roll onto her stomach, even in sleep. As a result, the back of her head was quite flat, and the sides appeared "pointy." Additionally, Ella's legs were stiff, she held her breath during certain movements, and she had difficulty sleeping.

Sandy Prantl: Ella's early intervention specialist was concerned about stiffness in Ella's legs and thought there may be a connection between her heart surgery and the stiffness she found. The therapist thought that CST might be helpful to correct this.

I evaluated Ella on January 21, 2003. Susan expressed additional concern about Ella's difficulty sleeping. Ella was reported to awaken several times per night. She presented with flexion habitus, sphenoid compression and inferior vertical strain lesions, tightness in her falx cerebelli, flattened nasal bones, and cranial base compression. Absence of cranial rhythm around the surgical site was also noted.

Susan: In the beginning, at the start of each session, Ella would roll around on the table and try to push away Sandy's hands. This was a bit stressful to me at first. Later, Ella was able to relax to the point of falling asleep. After a few sessions, she was sleeping for longer intervals during the night and taking naps during the day.

Sandy: In a session on April 8, 2003, I placed my hands on Ella's chest and melded with her. I silently asked her how I could help. Ella was worried about how her mommy and daddy were going to handle her situation. She related that the purpose of this experience was to "teach Mommy to be brave." During that time, the surgical scar and surrounding tissue softened and relaxed, and the cranial rhythm restarted in that area.

Susan: I sensed something more than usual was going on during that session. Ella was visibly upset. She wasn't trying to roll or get away, just crying and wringing her hands. I'm grateful that Sandy shared with me what she saw going on.

Ella, being only two, cannot yet verbalize her feelings about the CST experience. As her mother, I can say I feel blessed. I don't know where Ella would be had we not taken the advice to seek CST. Sandy has said about Ella, "She finds what she needs." In this instance, I'm sure glad she did.

Sandy: Ella's course of CranioSacral Therapy resolved the stiffness in her extremities and her sleep problems, and it "normalized" the shape of her head. She has developed normally using a combination of CST and conventional therapy methods.

This family is special to me in that Ella was clear about the life lessons her health problems had to teach her and her family. It is also a privilege to know Susan, who has been so open to Ella's healing process and the challenges to "being brave" that she has faced.

Susan M. Hartung, Ella's Mom,
and
Sandra Prantl, OTR/L, CST-D
Cincinnati, Ohio
CranioSacral Therapy Practitioner since 1992

Hope Rises Out of Tragedy

✿ At the age of six months, Mikey* suffered a near-fatal shaken-baby incident at the hands of his babysitter. He sustained multiple injuries that included a skull fracture, severe brain trauma, and several broken ribs. Life hung in the balance for days. Even if he were to survive, a bleak quality of life was expected.

Placed in a therapeutic coma for two weeks, Mikey emerged with severe spastic quadriplegia, cortical blindness, loss of auditory responses, and cognitive impairments. He also required a gastrostomy tube for nutritional support. Following three months of hospitalization, he was discharged home.

Over the next eight months, Mikey's functional improvements were very minimal, despite intense physical, occupational, and speech therapies. His rehab team members recommended a trial of Cranio-Sacral Therapy (CST).

It was now fourteen months since his injury. Mikey was twenty months of age and functioning at or below zero to three months of age in all areas, except for oral motor control, which was at four to six months.

Mikey presented with numerous problems. His arms were held in tight flexion. His hands were fisted. His head was constantly twisted toward the right shoulder. He displayed seizure-like activity. He had cortical blindness. Both eyes were deviated off midline and didn't focus. His optic nerves showed little to no response to light. He was unable to sleep restfully, waking eight to ten times every night in a distressed state. His vocalizations were high-pitched and consistent with brain trauma. He was easily startled by environmental stimuli and difficult to console once distressed. He remained in a chronic sympathetic nervous system state of over-arousal. And this wasn't everything.

---

*Name changed to protect client confidentiality

Craniosacral system assessment revealed a severely restricted, shortened dural tube. Three of the meningeal layers felt adhered to each other. The lines of fascial pull were so great that it felt like Mikey's buttocks were being pulled toward the back of his skull. The cranial vault felt stretched from internal pressure, and there was no palpable craniosacral rhythm at any point on the skull. Craniosacral rhythm was detected only in the lower legs, though it was diminished in amplitude and quality. His lumbosacral junction was immobile. Mikey became highly distressed whenever the occipital cranial base was palpated, as well as any time he was laid on his back.

Treatment began with one-hour sessions, twice a week. Our first session was essentially a long series of rock-and-glide techniques to support and reduce tension through the dural tube. Mikey could not tolerate any touch to his head.

At Mikey's next appointment, his parents reported that he had not had any seizures. There was also a very noticeable increase in his head control. In this session I detected a great degree of tissue tightness throughout the left side of his entire body, cranial nerve pathways, dural tube, and surrounding structures. I applied a cranial base release and sustained dural tube traction along with a parietal lift and frontal lift. Mikey was a bit more tolerant of touch to the head. By the end of the session, his muscle tone had dramatically relaxed.

By the next week, Mikey's parents reported that he had slept through the night for the first time since the accident, and that the quality of his sleep was deeper and more restful. No seizure activity, either.

Our next session started with dural tube elongation, both from the sacrum and the cranial base. I then proceeded to a good deal of cranial work with sphenoid decompression.

At our fourth session, the sphenoid decompression held for fifty minutes. Mikey's muscle tone was significantly reducing at rest, though still increasing when his position moved. There was enough reduction in spasticity to allow for voluntary kicking motion on his left side, like he was riding a bicycle. On the home front, Mikey was heard laughing and was easier to calm and console.

With more therapy, Mikey was able to lie on the table without distress for an entire hour. He frequently laughed, giggled, and cooed. His legs were beginning to move separately from each other and less reflexively. Following one particular week, Mikey experienced a spontaneous reenactment of his birth. He actively pulled himself into a fetal position several times and rested there for quite a while. For a body with spastic quadriplegia to do this is just short of miraculous.

Many other changes began to occur in Mikey as well. When a brightly lit ball was placed on his lap, he pulled himself forward to look at it. This was the first true visual response he had shown since his injury. Today, his eyes move together consistently and constantly.

Mikey has regained ninety to ninety-five percent of his head control, and it no longer lists to the right. His parents can carry him with greater ease since the spasticity has reduced by eighty to ninety percent. His arms have relaxed out of spastic flexion posturing when he is not being moved. And he can now respond very quickly to efforts to calm him when he becomes distressed.

Another surprise in all this is that Mikey's reflux problem, which he had had since birth, disappeared with the CST. His parents have been able to take him off all medications for that.

Mikey has a long way to go to maximize his recovery from this trauma, but his entire rehabilitation team is convinced that his progress to date is directly related to the addition of CranioSacral Therapy. His parents, though remaining realistic about the future, are amazed at the "unexplained" rate and percentage of recovery their son has gained in such a short period of time. Their optimism and intention to guide their son out of the darkness have surely supported his own spirit and inner drive toward recovery.

Susan Vaughan Kratz, OTR, BCP
Waukesha, Wisconsin
CranioSacral Therapy Practitioner since 2000

The Face of Gratitude

Last year my granddaughter's mother, Tina, gave birth to her fifth child, a baby girl named Azurée. The birth was somewhat difficult, as Azurée's head was a bit large.

I noticed immediately that this child was different from her sister. She slept a lot and was not very animated. She would smile when spoken to but seemed to be lethargic most of the time. The doctors were worried about her head being too big and thought she might have hydrocephalus. At five months she began to pull at her ear and would scream for ten to fifteen minutes. This would occur several times a week. The doctors gave her antibiotics for a so-called ear infection, but the problem persisted.

I talked with Tina about seeing a friend of mine who did pediatric CranioSacral Therapy (CST). I set up an appointment with Ben McClung, who is an excellent therapist and very good with babies. We placed Azurée on the massage table, and Ben began his assessment of her.

Azurée tried to look up and around at him to see what he was doing, but she didn't cry. Ben turned her so that she could see what he was doing. He felt her atlanto-occipital joint and noted that it was severely compressed. We sat her up and Ben gently placed two fingers in that area and began applying CST.

Azurée immediately began crying hard. Sweat began forming on her head, and the area was very hot according to Ben. He continued for about three minutes, and then Tina asked him to stop because she didn't like hearing her baby cry. Ben took his hand away, and Azurée stopped crying. She sat there for a few minutes and then smiled at Ben, grabbed his face, pulled him toward her, and put her mouth on his cheek. It was the most amazing expression of gratitude I have ever seen in my practice.

Ben saw Azurée once more after that, and the problems stopped. Her head is now of normal size and, at thirteen months of age, she is a pistol—inquisitive, verbal, and walking. The pain she experienced earlier is gone. I feel blessed to have witnessed this and am very grateful for John Upledger and the courses he provides.

Over the years Ben and I have worked together with many people, but this was the first time I worked with a baby. I found the experience extremely rewarding.

Jeanne Elsen, LMT, NCTMB
Albuquerque, New Mexico
CranioSacral Therapy Practitioner since 1993

CST Accelerates Progress

✿ Shortly after my first CranioSacral Therapy course in August 2002, I began treating Baby K.* The experience not only changed my perception of the body and its capacity to heal, but had an extraordinary effect on my view of myself as an occupational therapist. This was the first time I had seen such significant changes in a child's system.

Baby K's diagnosis was severe right torticollis. Mom had initial concerns regarding her baby's lack of head and arm control, as well as her very weak cry. She also reported that the baby spit up following eating, was somewhat irritable, and had difficulty sleeping through the night.

I started seeing Baby K when she was four months old. What I saw was a baby not only with tightness in her neck but restrictions in every part of her existence. I utilized the ELAP (Early Learning Accomplishment Profile) as part of my evaluation. This profile looks at gross motor, fine motor, language, and cognitive skills. Baby K scored consistently at a newborn to one-month level in all areas except cognition, which went up to two months. She was unable to lift her head in a prone position (on her stomach) for more than one or two seconds. She preferred being on her back.

Baby K made only one sound besides her weak cry, and that was a grunting noise. This concerned me. This baby had increased stiffness on her left side and very limited active movement of her left arm. She would smile but was only able to utilize the lower portion of her face. She also lacked active movement of her arms and legs. She was unable to fully rotate her head from left to right when she was held upright. She appeared to be stuck in an active alert state. And Mom reported that she slept poorly during the day and at nighttime.

---

*Name omitted to protect client confidentiality

I began treating Baby K one hour per week with CranioSacral Therapy. At first her craniosacral rhythm was dull and underactive, with decreased symmetry, quality, amplitude, and rate, and her system was resistant to treatment. Then releases started to occur more easily and naturally.

Each week Baby K had significant improvements, and I repeated all the release techniques I learned in the CST class, except those for the cranial bones. I wanted to do the cranial bone releases when I had gained more experience with this approach.

I gave Mom some oral motor activities to try at home to help stimulate Baby K's mouth movement and control. The next time we would meet, Mom would always say, "I don't know what you did but ..."

Baby K's first big change was in her cry. Mom said, "I'm not sure if I should thank you or not!" After one week of therapy she had developed a very loud cry along with improved head rotation and control. This baby began bringing her hands together and started to roll. As her arm control improved, she would greet me by touching my face or arm. I found that amazing.

Baby K had decreased stiffness and improved quality/symmetry of movement. Her smile broadened, and her grunting decreased. Within a few weeks she was making a variety of sounds. She was also able to regulate her states. She was more relaxed and demonstrated improved sleeping patterns.

Within eight weeks of her initial evaluation, Baby K was age-appropriate in all areas of the ELAP. She had gained four months' worth of skills in less than four months. The physical therapist noticed all the changes and said to me, "Teach me everything you are doing."

Baby K's orthopedist discharged her from his services. He told her mom that it usually takes longer than a year to reach this level of improvement. And her pediatrician said that the therapy had excellent success and was well worth it.

By January 2003, Baby K's occupational and physical therapy

appointments were down to once a month. She was soon discharged completely. At seven months of age, she began crawling forward, and at eleven months was almost walking. I later taught Mom some infant massage techniques, which she used on a daily basis.

Baby K's progress was no doubt related to CranioSacral Therapy, her family's excellent follow-through with infant massage, and all the other suggested home activities.

In April 2003 I was invited to present this case on a panel at the Beyond the Dura research conference in Florida. This experience has opened my mind and heart to the possibilities of CranioSacral Therapy.

Corinne Eckley, OTR/L
Arnold, Maryland
CranioSacral Therapy Practitioner since 2002

An Angelle Changed My Life

My story begins with the birth of my third child, Angelle Elizabeth, born on February 18, 1995. Angelle was born with craniosynostosis, chronic static encephalopathy, and mild cerebral palsy. She was extremely different-looking as a baby due to the premature fusing of her right lambdoidal suture and three-fourths of her saggital.

Angelle was diagnosed with brain injury at eight months of age and craniosynostosis when she was two years old. She was extremely mentally and physically delayed. When she was one year old we started her in an intensive program that included physical therapy, occupational therapy, speech therapy, and work with a special teacher. It involved a one-hundred-and-twenty-mile drive two days a week. This went on for two and a half years, until Angelle went into the Three to Six program in the public school system.

Angelle had a problem retrieving information from her brain and using it again when needed. Her syndrome was causing her jaws to be pushed to the left side of her face and her head to become very misshapen. She was in a great deal of pain. She had cluster migraine headaches when she was five years old.

I was introduced to CranioSacral Therapy (CST) by our family chiropractor and decided to study the technique myself. I started working with Angelle when she was four years old.

I can tell you firsthand the changes that took place in my little girl. She began to retrieve information quicker and was able to function better. She had a movement disorder, which became eighty percent better with CST. She advanced so much in her learning that she became top of her special class when she was five years old.

Angelle could follow two- and three-step commands without hesitating, which she had been unable to do in the past. Her language skills improved. When she entered first grade she no longer needed speech therapy, and by the end of second grade no longer needed occupational therapy.

Angelle has not had one migraine headache since she was five and a half years old. With the intraoral work I do, her jaw has maintained and not gotten any worse. Her doctors have been amazed with her progress. Her neurologist could not believe how the migraines stopped with the CranioSacral Therapy. In fact, he was fascinated by the work.

Angelle is now going into fourth grade and is in the regular classroom, with the exception of math classes; she has a mild learning disability in this subject.

I know in my heart that had we not found CranioSacral Therapy, Angelle's life story may not have had such a wonderful ending.

Julie Wachter
Prairie du Chien, Wisconsin
CranioSacral Therapy Practitioner since 2003

Brothers Take Charge of Lives

❀ I had the opportunity to work with two brothers, ages sixteen and twenty, who had been diagnosed with Tourette's syndrome. The particular concern of each was eye twitching, which affected them when they were in social and public situations, such as dates and choral performances.

Through CranioSacral Therapy we worked on releasing their stress and symptoms. Working individually with each young man, I followed the cranial rhythm to where his body pulled me in to listen more deeply. I was able to gently feel releases under my fingers as each brother experienced some very deep releases from his whole body.

The older brother was amazed at how quickly he stopped twitching after the first session. During our second session, he told me that when he felt the twitching surface, he was able to step back and stop or at least control it.

The younger brother would get headaches, and we were able to free him from the pressure as well as control his eye twitching. He said that he even tried some of the techniques on himself, and they worked on numerous occasions.

These young men are very happy with the cranial work and continue to receive treatments as necessary. The younger brother has just graduated from high school and is going on to college to become a pharmacist. The older brother just graduated from college and is going on to law school.

The utilization of CranioSacral Therapy illustrates the benefits that can be derived. It also shows, in this instance, how it allowed two young men to embrace the opportunity to take charge of their own lives.

Jocelyn Pare, MEd
Alameda, California
CranioSacral Therapy Practitioner since 1991

Palate Perfect

❀ In 2000 I moved from the East Coast to the Midwest with my teenage daughter. In her anger over the move, she managed to physically alter the structure of her upper palate so that her teeth, which were in perfect alignment before the move, were now misaligned and causing her serious headaches. There was no bruxism or TMJ syndrome. She had caused this alteration over a four-month period.

Doctors at the University of Michigan School of Dentistry wanted to break her jaw and reconstruct it. I didn't consider this a viable option, and so I set about researching alternatives. Having been in massage therapy for a number of years, I remembered reading about CranioSacral Therapy and its use with such conditions. I signed up for a class.

Upon completion of the CranioSacral Therapy course, I waited a few weeks and then did a 10-Step Protocol on my daughter. She fell asleep while I worked on her, but woke up yelling at me, as her entire face had snapped loudly during the sphenoid decompression. Her bite was immediately perfect, and I was a very happy mom. I use CranioSacral Therapy in my practice all the time now.

Joanne Scott, LMT
Ann Arbor, Michigan
CranioSacral Therapy Practitioner since 2000

"I Lost My Brave"

✿ There it was, Kyle's name on the emergencies-only kids slot on my schedule. I wondered what was going on. He knew to tell his mom when it was time to come back to see me for another session. Curiosity filled my thoughts as I prepared for his visit.

Kyle and I went back a long way. It had been more than seven years since we began CranioSacral Therapy (CST) together. What an outrageous soul this one was. It was amazing that he was still alive.

When I first saw Kyle he was twenty-two months old. Born prematurely, he had spent his first thirty-seven days of life on a respirator. The official diagnosis was chylothorax hydrops. This involved excessive fluid in the pleural cavities, which necessitated chest tubes for drainage. He was small for his age, with skinny little arms and legs. He had a full head of brilliant red hair and eyes that were dark, almost black. His belly was hard and distended; his breathing was shallow; and he had difficulty swallowing. A feeding tube and a central line were in place. His mother stated that he had endured more than three hundred X-rays in his short life. The latest diagnosis was leukemia.

In the weeks and months that followed, Kyle underwent rounds and rounds of chemotherapy and frequent spinal taps. The intravenous ports were often infected, requiring replacements. There was continual stomach distress, trouble with antibiotics, numerous hospitalizations for septic blood infections, feeding tube difficulties, and struggles with learning how to swallow and take food orally. The challenges went on and on. Yet, finally, the leukemia was in remission, and he had made it to his sixth birthday.

A couple of months later, however, the leukemia was back. There was more radiation, more chemotherapy and, this time, a stem-cell transplant. Again, success.

Through all this, CranioSacral Therapy was vital to Kyle's journey. At our very first session, a huge amount of what I considered to be "terror energy" had been released from his body. His eyes literally changed from almost black to an orange/green color. Sessions were often weekly, scheduled the day after chemotherapy, spinal taps, or other hospitalizations.

Kyle's body always told me exactly what to do. As time went by, he could even verbalize the place in his body that needed the most work. In reviewing his chart, I noticed that every session demanded a considerable amount of time working on the bones. I also noted that he "rallied well" with CranioSacral Therapy.

His whole family benefited from CST over time. When Mom couldn't handle the pressure anymore, when dad's back hurt so badly he couldn't stand up straight, when little sister would scream through the night—all were comforted and supported with CranioSacral Therapy.

Fast forward to the day of Kyle's "emergency" visit. Now nine years old, he was accompanied by his mother and four-year-old sister. Mom explained that the whole family had been dealing with the flu. Exhausted, Mom and Sister quickly found the big pillows and blanket in my office and promptly lay down on the floor of my therapy room.

Kyle climbed on the massage table and tearfully whispered, "I lost my brave." He told how the whole family had gotten the flu and was throwing up. He was terrified to sleep in his own bed. He was frantic and his stomach was in spasm.

I let him know that there had been more than a couple times in my life that I, too, had "lost my brave." With this I invited him to get really quiet, and together we set about finding his "brave." As the session progressed I reminded him of all the times he had been brave facing all sorts of challenges.

I continually asked Kyle's body to release all the scared feelings that might still be there. It was a deeply quiet session, and my hands never left his abdomen. Forty-five minutes later, he sat up and said, "That's a lot better." With that he hopped off the table, woke up

his mom and sister, helped them gather their belongings, and con-
fidently walked out the door.

Kyle is thriving in regular school now; he's in the third grade.
All the tubes are out of his body, and medical check-ups are needed
less and less. He is off all medication with the exception of growth
hormone shots.

What a profound reminder. We all lose our "brave" sometimes.
It's comforting to know that CranioSacral Therapy is a very safe
place to find it again.

Evy O'Leary, RN, LCPC
Missoula, Montana
CranioSacral Therapy Practitioner since 1991

Latching On and Making Up for Lost Time

Marie was four days old when I saw her for the first time. She was the third child for this couple. Labor had been short, and delivery unmedicated and complication-free, as it had been with each prior child.

While still in the hospital, the experienced mother was helping her roommate with the early difficulties of breastfeeding when she realized that her own new baby was not latching on at all. Hungry and needing that closeness to her mother, Marie grew more frustrated by the day. Mom was worried and disappointed. How could she have failed after successfully breastfeeding two other babies?

It was during a home visit that the mother's lactation advisor recommended CranioSacral Therapy to help Marie latch on better. That's when I entered the picture.

I was surprised to see Marie's little face. Not only was she frustrated and hungry, but her nose was angled off to one side and her chin to the other, making her look like she was slightly deformed. Her cranial and facial bones were so out of position that I could barely get my finger into her mouth to feel the palate. There was no room at all between the tongue and palate. This tightness did not allow the tongue to move or the jaw to drop in order to latch on to the breast properly.

It was close to an hour before Marie decided to go with the program. Her frustration was so great that she had no interest in anyone doing anything other than feeding her. She wanted food—and she couldn't get it. The parents tried a bottle, but Marie could not move her tongue to suck.

Finally, as Marie began to relax, Mom quietly asked me if I could see what was happening. Marie's nose was slowly beginning to move back toward the center line of her little face. It sent chills down my back to see her nose inching into proper position. Once it stopped, I moved my finger from her mouth to see if we could encourage the jaw to do the same. This didn't take nearly as much time. Marie already knew how to do this, and her little jaw settled into position.

Marie's face now looked relaxed and symmetrical, and she was given yet another chance to get some food. Breathing excitedly, she moved her little head quickly from side to side trying to find the nipple. Remembering that she couldn't do this, she dropped her head back and screamed with frustration. It must have seemed like a bad tease: knowing where the food was but unable to get any.

After repeated attempts, Marie's jaw suddenly dropped low and Mom quickly got the nipple into her mouth. This time it was perfect! At first Marie sucked very slowly, as if she were testing the possibilities. Soon realizing that she was getting milk this time, Marie became a machine, making up for lost time.

Ilona E. Trommler, LMT
Westlake, Ohio
CranioSacral Therapy Practitioner since 1998

Babies Benefit from Gentle Releases

❀ I had been a massage therapist for about two years when I decided to take CranioSacral Therapy, levels one and two. I was thrilled beyond words during the classes. This form of bodywork struck me so deeply that I had dreams about it night after night.

I recalled that a long time before then, after graduating from college and moving to Colorado to find my "adult" self, I visited an elder wise woman who was very intuitive. I was a professional counselor struggling with my own direction and life purpose. This woman foresaw me doing a very rare and different type of massage or bodywork in the future. She didn't have a name for it, but said I would find great meaning in it and that it would affect my life profoundly. That was 1982.

Sitting in a CranioSacral Therapy class in 1996, I realized that this was exactly what she had been talking about all those years ago. Chills ran up my spine.

While managing a spa in Wisconsin, I met a woman who was a foster-care mother. She and her husband took care of babies during their transition from the natural mother to adoptive parents. She nurtured these little ones for a few days, a few weeks, or a few months, depending on their placement schedule. Upon learning that I was a massage therapist, she asked if I would do bodywork on them. My gift was the opportunity to do CranioSacral Therapy on these infants. It was an incredible and delightful experience to watch and feel the transition and transformation in these babies as they released what they needed to at that time. I hoped, in some small way, to help these children with their birth trauma and their adoptive process. Maybe their bodies and souls would be a bit more integrated after having this gentle and loving bodywork, and their lives more positive because of it. That was my intention, and we know intention is very significant.

Having gained some experience with babies, I gathered the

courage one holiday season during a family visit to ask my niece Tara if I could work on her baby daughter Kiera, who had colic.

After three months of nightly cries, not only was the baby miserable, but new mom Tara was pale and frail. My husband Rob and I exchanged knowing glances as she explained the frustration and helplessness she felt. When she briefly left the room I asked Rob what he thought about me doing CranioSacral Therapy on Kiera. He looked at me with the unspoken thought of "It's time to come out of the alternative-therapy closet."

I had that fluttery, step-out-of-the-comfort-zone feeling that we therapists experience when trying to explain what we do to people who know absolutely nothing about this work and are skeptical about anything beyond their normal realm of existence. This family unit was definitely from that mold. Thus, Rob and I had shared little of our knowledge on these subjects.

When we asked permission, a brief pause filled the room, followed by a definitive "Yes" from Tara. I had already silently asked the little one, Kiera, if it was okay for me to do bodywork on her.

The whole family was gathered in the living room watching. I stepped to the couch and talked to Kiera. Even though she was only three months old, I believe children understand and comprehend a great deal more than we realize. Out of respect for her, I wanted her to know what I was going to do.

Whenever I start a bodywork session, I call on angels and guides to be present for protection, balance, and healing. It is part of my protocol. It sets the tone and resonance for the session. As I requested this silently to myself, Kiera broke into a huge smile. When I noticed her reaction, I whispered, "Kiera, can you see the angels?" She was staring above my head, as babies do. She smiled again. I was struck by the wisdom and knowing of this three-month-old. Tears welled up in my eyes.

I did an infant still point. She became very quiet, still, and serious. I worked on her mid-back and stomach area. Her diaphragm released. She squirmed, wiggled, and giggled. The session lasted about ten minutes. Then, suddenly, I knew she was ready to be done. She turned her head and smiled again, while her eyes held something I couldn't see above my head. I knew she was sensing things I could only imagine. The family paid us little attention during this time. I gently transferred Kiera to her mom. She smiled at me with gratitude and hope. Rob and I glanced at each other again, knowing the healing had happened.

About two weeks after we visited, Tara called to let us know that the colic was gone. It had been gone since the day I worked on Kiera. Mom, Dad, and Baby were sleeping peacefully every night. I was overjoyed and deeply grateful. Words cannot express the power and healing of CranioSacral Therapy. My exalted dream is to have every baby born on this planet experience it.

Kim Kee, MT
Sault Ste Marie, Michigan
CranioSacral Therapy Practitioner since 1996

Problems Traced Decade Later to Birth Trauma

❀ A co-worker and client of mine with multiple sclerosis told me during one of our weekly sessions that she had referred one of her friends, also a co-worker, to me in the hopes that I might be able to help her daughter.

The next day at work, I contacted this lady, who said she had tried everything to help her ten-year-old daughter Melissa, who had been diagnosed ADD/ADHD and been on and off numerous drugs, including Ritalin.

This mother was at her wits' end. She was fighting with the school principal and doctors, who wanted to put her daughter back on Ritalin or have her transferred to a special facility for kids with learning disabilities and social dysfunction. Their reasons were many. Melissa was socially withdrawn and introverted, yet experienced bouts of severe mood swings. She was very uncoordinated and often teased by the other kids. Her speech was slurred. Her mental processes were delayed at best. She had constant headaches and chronic ear infections. It was impossible for her to stay focused for more than twenty or thirty minutes at a time. And she was failing or near failing almost all of her classes.

While talking with the mother in her office, I noticed a picture of Melissa taped to her computer monitor. It showed a striking asymmetry between the left and right sides of Melissa's face from midline. The right side of her face was twice as wide as the left, and I was unable to see the left ear when looking straight at her from the front. When I brought this to the mother's attention, she was shocked and stated that she had never noticed it before, as she had never known Melissa to be any other way. Upon further questioning, I learned that Melissa's delivery was extremely difficult. It had lasted over fifteen hours and culminated with a suction birth that was wrought with high drama and tension. We made an appointment.

When Melissa arrived for her CranioSacral Therapy (CST) session, she was the epitome of a hyperactive kid. After the formalities were out of the way, I got Melissa on the table and checked her for a leg-length discrepancy. I found her to be approximately one-half inch longer on the left side, which I corrected quickly using simple isometric techniques. I then balanced her pelvic and respiratory diaphragms, getting quite a bit of movement with both. When I started a thoracic opening release, her neck immediately started to release and unwind. I then went to a CV-4 technique, which dropped her into an immediate still point and put her to sleep.

What happened next brings tears to my eyes every time I think about it. Upon positioning my hands to do a frontal lift, I noticed a very pronounced ridge at the coronal suture. It seems that the suction device used during childbirth had caused lifting of the parietal bones to the extent that the frontal bone dropped down and the parietal ridge came to rest on top of it. This greatly stretched the fascial membrane between the fronto-parietal suture. I couldn't even comprehend the enormous pressures and forces this must have been exerting over the ten-year lifetime of this child. It's no wonder she was having so many problems!

As I started the lift, an enormous rush of pain and anguish swept over me as we moved through release after release. Suddenly it was as if we had moved mountains. Everything let go, and it felt as if I had lifted her frontal bone three to four inches. In fact, it was closer to six to eight millimeters, as the two parietal bones moved back into their normal position. This one release lasted almost twelve minutes. After it was through, the ridge was gone and Melissa's fronto-parietal junction was completely smooth.

I then did a parietal lift, which brought on yet another wave of dark pain and anguish. After things settled down, I moved to the mastoid wobble, temporal rotation, and ear pull to finish out the session.

Throughout the whole session, Melissa was experiencing rapid eye movement. She remarked after she woke up a few minutes later that she had just had the most beautiful dream ever. The most remarkable part was that after just one forty-five-minute session, complete symmetry had returned to her face and head. Both her mother and I were completely amazed that the human body could do something so profound.

A couple of weeks later, Mom stopped me in the hall to say that Melissa's principal had called her and said, "What did you do to Melissa? She's a totally different person!" Mom reported back to me at the end of the semester that Melissa had made her first A in school and that she was now a solid B and C student for the first time in her life. She was no longer considered ADD/ADHD. She was getting along with all of her classmates. She was enrolled in Kung Fu classes and was doing very well with her hand/eye coordination skills. In addition, her speech impediment had all but cleared up. She told me that Melissa was calling me her hero!

Shortly after that, our company was bought out in a merger and we were forced to go our separate ways, but I ran into the both of them a couple of years later. Melissa was a beautiful young lady who was now a black belt in Kung Fu, an above-average kid in school, and had not had an ear infection since our first session together. I call her my miracle girl!

Any doubts I may ever have had about the efficacy of CST were eliminated that fateful day when I held that young girl's head in my hands and was privileged to be part of a true miracle. Thank you, Dr. John, for having the courage to elevate CST to the level you have. The world will never be the same!

Chuck Olson, RMT
Bellville, Texas
CranioSacral Therapy Practitioner since 1998

CST and a Root Canal

When I was in college, I wanted to change the world. I thought that meant law school, until my own health problems led me in a new direction. Unable to find help for my allergies, migraines, and depression, I began looking beyond mainstream medicine for solutions. Professionally I went into the healing arts, becoming a midwife and then a registered massage therapist. Personally, my search to heal myself eventually led me to CranioSacral Therapy (CST).

It was this knowledge that benefited my son Wiley when, at the age of eight years, he broke his tooth when he ran into a brick wall while playing ball. It was a scary and very painful time for him. This incident challenged/pushed me as a practitioner because I had to put aside my personal fears and maternal anxieties to help him. I have sometimes felt frustrated because, although I can do all these great processes with my clients, I have been too emotionally close to help my own children.

Our pediatric dentist X-rayed Wiley's tooth and said he would need a root canal. Not willing to accept that, I took his X-rays to a holistic dentist for a second opinion. He also recommended a root canal. When I questioned him, he revealed that any signs of infection would be evident as inflammation, pain, and/or fever.

I had heard horror stories about root canals and was firm that my little boy was not to be subjected to one. I felt he was too young to understand, and I wanted to protect him from that trauma. My three children have rarely experienced any kind of medical intervention, and I aim to keep it that way!

I decided that, despite the urgent promptings of the dentists, we would wait and see. Our pediatric dentist gained my affection and respect because she agreed to stand by, monitor the tooth, and advise me over time.

I pursued CranioSacral Therapy. Initially I took him to a Cranio-

Sacral Therapist proficient at working in the mouth, since I had not yet reached that level in my studies. Gradually, however, as I studied Advanced CST and beyond, I began working on Wiley myself once in a while.

Six years passed. Finally, in the fall of 2003, after taking a look at Wiley's X-rays, our dentist said, "It's time." By then Wiley was fifteen, and I felt he could handle a root canal, and I could handle him having one. We scheduled with an endodontist.

The night before his appointment, I took Wiley to my studio for CranioSacral Therapy. I held the injured tooth to let it unwind. It was bouncing all over the place. I heard a little helpless voice, shouting in a panic, "Don't hurt me, don't hurt me, don't hurt me!" I held the tooth gently, and it gradually became calm and quiet.

I gave the tooth some time to settle down and enjoy these changes. Then I talked to the tissues, telling them in some detail what would happen during the root canal. I reassured them that Wiley would be safe throughout the procedure.

The next morning I took Wiley to the endodontist. After witnessing the prep, I retired to the waiting room. Despite my best efforts to trust and relax, I was tense. I sat and prayed.

Afterward, Wiley felt only minor discomfort from having his jaw open so long. Driving home, he said to me, "I think these things are going to be really terrible, but then when I go through them, it's no big deal."

Later, as I was reflecting on the experience, I realized that the little panicky voice saying, "Don't hurt me!" sounded like *my* voice.

I believe my own fears and anxieties at the time of the accident when Wiley was eight had "jumped" from my nervous system into his tissues. I had seen this phenomenon in [Dr. Upledger's] "The Brain Speaks" class and also in my private practice. Wiley's pain and fear coupled with our close bond had created an entryway for my anxieties to invade his tissues.

With CranioSacral Therapy, his body dropped its resistance and fears. Who can say what his experience would have been had he undergone treatment with the tooth area being highly agitated. Certainly the potential for complications and inflammation would have been much greater. The endodontist would have had to struggle with a tooth that was vibrating at a micro level in total panic, trying to evade his ministrations. Those movements would have given him a moving target instead of a calm, steady ground.

The endodontist did mention he had some difficulties with the root of the tooth, due to Wiley's youthful age at the time of the accident. He also said it was much better that we had waited until now.

My son went to school the next day. He didn't miss a step. He felt *no* pain.

The funniest part was that, with all of my "positive thinking," the *one* outcome that never occurred to me was this perfect outcome. I am grateful for the huge lesson I received in trust and faith.

Nancy Kern, RMT, MFA
Houston, Texas
CranioSacral Therapy Practitioner since 1998

No Helmet for Henry

When we first met Henry, he was about five months old. His mother, initially a bit apprehensive, was quickly won over by the rapid results achieved by CranioSacral Therapy. Following is what she wrote about the experience.

"Ever since my baby, Henry, could turn over, he had a preference for sleeping on his right side. This resulted, at the age of about two to three months, in a flattening on the back of his head and a consequent bulging at the front. He could not be persuaded to sleep on his left side. His craniofacial asymmetry worsened to the point where the ear on his right side was shifted forward. The pediatrician recommended a craniofacial examination.

"After we waited anxiously for almost two months for an approval from my insurance company, Henry was evaluated. The report stated severe bilateral occipital flattening, or brachycephaly, along with severe fronto-temporal flattening and an anterior shift of his right ear, orbit, and cranial base. The pediatric craniofacial orthotist stated that Henry required a dynamic orthotic cranioplasty (DOC), a kind of headband or helmet that the baby was to wear twenty-three hours a day.

"I was horrified! Even as an adult who understands, I couldn't conceive of going through the process of having the plaster mold made and then wearing the helmet for twenty-three hours a day, sleeping and eating in it. So what would it be like for my sweet baby boy?

"I was told that any delay in treatment would allow a progression of the asymmetries. I was very concerned, since I knew that the bones of his head were hardening day by day. I did not want his head to stay this way or get worse.

"There just had to be another way. A friend of mine confided to me that her son had experienced cranial problems as a baby, and that CranioSacral Therapy from Dr. Diane Sandler had helped him. I had to make a big decision. I finally determined to go with 'a mother's gut feeling'—a big gamble considering it was my son's future at stake.

"Henry was treated by Dr. Sandler, Charlene Papazian, and Porche Lottermoser once a week. The treatment was probably more exhausting for me than for Henry, since, as a mother, I have a very hard time listening to my baby cry.

"Henry worked out many issues: his birth ten days early, his cesarean delivery, three months of colic, and horrid teething pain. At first, doubts would creep into my mind as I saw him crying. 'Am I doing the right thing?' I wondered. I was! The results were immediate.

"After each treatment there was a visible, major improvement that continued for days after. Within a few months we could stretch the treatments from every two weeks to every four weeks.

"By the time Henry turned one year old, his head was beautifully round and normal-looking. The pediatricians were very surprised, since they were only familiar with the DOC treatment, but they admitted, 'The result speaks for itself.'

"Around that time, Henry also started walking. We stopped the treatments at that point because it was hard to keep up with a toddler. I am returning today for a general CranioSacral treatment. Henry is now eighteen months old and can always benefit from the therapy.

"Henry and I are eternally grateful to Dr. Sandler and her assistants, Charlene and Porche."

Sylvia A.

Diane Sandler, LAc, OMD, CST-D
Toluca Lake, California
CranioSacral Therapy Practitioner since 1993

Charlene Papazian, LMT, CST
Toluca Lake, California
CranioSacral Therapy Practitioner since 2001

Porche Lottermoser, CMT
Glendale, California
CranioSacral Therapy Practitioner since 2001

Is Benign Really Harmless?

❁ The first time I saw twenty-four-month-old Hanna, she presented with a number of problems, including ADHD, verbal delay, coordination problems (including several falls), and large emotional swings. She also experienced bouts of little or no appetite, lethargy, and occasional nausea, according to her mother. Her diagnosis was benign hydrocephalus. The medical opinion for this patient was: "Leave the condition alone; she may grow out of it."

Hanna's mother brought her to me after researching Cranio-Sacral Therapy on the Internet and deciding to "give it a try."

At our initial visit, it was evident from Hanna's shrieks of discontent that she didn't like the idea of a stranger doing any kind of hands-on assessment. This behavior lasted through about three treatments. Then, with the help of Mom and the right toys, Hanna became a little more comfortable with the situation.

When I was finally able to evaluate Hanna, her craniosacral rhythm seemed quite stagnant, showing little movement from full flexion to neutral. Total vibrancy seemed to be about twenty to thirty percent of full normal. Very gradually she allowed me to do some hands-on CranioSacral Therapy—still point induction and a modified CV-4. She was very resistant to work around the ears and temporals, as many children are.

Following six or seven treatments, Hanna was comfortable with most of the 10-Step Protocol and direction of energy techniques. We worked to enhance the motion of the dorsal tube as well as the amplitude and vibrancy of the craniosacral rhythm. The atlanto-occipito joint needed particular attention, and we applied greater lumbar compressions over that area.

Since starting CranioSacral Therapy, Hanna's sleeping schedule and appetite have normalized. Her behavior is more controlled. Her vocabulary has increased to over a hundred words. She is able to speak in short sentences. And she has not fallen except in certain normal play situations. Her mother still brings Hanna in when her appetite and energy wane. We will keep a watch on her during growth and development.

Richard G. Hofner, MS, PT, ATC, CST
Hamburg, New York
CranioSacral Therapy Practitioner since 1994

Bianca's Story

❁ I received a telephone call from Frank and Andrea Morales on June 29, 2003. They were desperately seeking help for their five-month-old daughter, Bianca, who had been born with a severely misshapen head.

They had received a report from their neurologist recommending that Bianca be put in a helmet for three or four years and possibly undergo surgery to remove part of the skull. At the time of the phone call, Bianca was awaiting an appointment to be fitted for a helmet.

Our first appointment was more or less a get-acquainted session. I observed that Bianca's head appeared to be twisted on at the top, like a jar lid, in a left-to-right direction, pushing the right frontal bone forward and elevating the parietal. Her right ear was forward and the left one back. In the back, there was a flattened three-inch area in the posterior temporal bone. The lower parietal on the left had an indentation you could lay your finger in. The posterior plates were overlapped and came to a point, protruding in the back.

I held Baby Bianca and did as much cranial work as I could with her tiny, squirming little body.

The next day, Mom reported that Bianca had slept through the night for the first time without waking for feeding. In this second session I gently massaged down either side of Bianca's spine. She let out a very large sigh, followed by another one a couple of minutes later. I felt we had witnessed two big releases.

When I saw Bianca a couple of days later, there was obvious physical change. Her cranial plates were moving! Rocking her in my arms, with my hand on the occiput, I felt two "clicks" in the cranium as the plates were correcting themselves, moving into sutural alignment after having been overlapped.

With Mom holding her, Bianca dropped her head down to her left shoulder, held it there a couple seconds, and then raised her chin toward the ceiling. After she had done this three times, I asked Mom if she had seen her do this before. She said no.

At our next appointment, Bianca showed profound changes to the cranium: It was smoother and there was softening.

Believing that the "twist" in the top portion of Bianca's head had also twisted the spine to the sacrum, I began the process of balancing the spine. I held one finger under the neck and held my other hand on the sacrum, "intending" gentle traction. Bianca fell asleep. I then did a parietal lift, which took about five minutes.

Suddenly, Bianca began to flail both arms and the right leg only. Her left leg was bent at the knee, with the heel right up to the butt. I had previously observed that she favored her left leg and was not able to maintain weight on it. I believed there was a blockage, an energy cyst of some sort, in Bianca's leg. As we continued to observe, the right leg continued to flail, and the arms were flapping up and down on the bed.

At this point, I moved away from Bianca and instructed Mom to stand back; the baby was self-correcting. Bianca would seem to awaken, look around, and shut her eyes again. She did this for a couple of minutes, then became fully awake. We were very excited and couldn't wait to see what would happen as time went on.

Over the next few months, Bianca continued to show wonderful improvements. Her head was rounding and filling out in the flattened areas. She was responding to toys. She was laughing at her three-year-old brother's attempts to gain her attention. She was sleeping through the night. There was more symmetry between the eyes. And she seemed much more at peace.

In mid-September Bianca had what I perceived as a major release in her spine and sacrum. Following a dural tube rock and parietal lift, there was an instant release of her left leg, and both legs literally flung straight out. From that point, she started to gain leg strength.

I continued working with Bianca through mid-October, when she was scheduled to be fitted for her helmet. By our final session, her face appeared more balanced. The back of her head was smoother and rounder. She could balance on both feet when held up by her fingers. She played the aggressor for the first time, reaching for my fingers and watch. And she loved to sing!

Thinking back to when I started doing CranioSacral Therapy (CST) on Bianca, I remember the family saying that they had tried to see her doctor to get his okay for CranioSacral Therapy, but were told he was too busy to see them. The next time they saw him was the day Bianca went for her helmet fitting. Looking at her, he insisted that the previous medical reports had to be impossible. When the Moraleses told him about the CST, he commented, "Oh, yeah, some of my patients do that. Keep it up."

I am happy to report that the helmet came off in three months. There was no surgery. And Bianca, now one year old, is even more beautiful.

The family had been told she would be developmentally slow—with everything from her teeth coming in to her motor skills. I can tell you that she walks, tries to run, and plays; is bright; has excellent motor skills; and her teeth are quickly filling in.

The family and I are thrilled and, we all agree, without Cranio-Sacral Therapy Bianca would still be in a helmet.

Thank you, Dr. John. Without you this would not have happened.

Jean A. Villmer, CMT
Bisbee, Arizona
CranioSacral Therapy Practitioner since 1997

Boy's Hip Dysfunction Eased with CST

❀ Several years ago I started treating a seven-year-old boy named Roger,* who had Perthes' disease of the hip. This is where the hip joint does not fit well into its capsule because it is flat instead of rounded. He had hip dysplasia at birth and wore rigid braces for the first few months. His doctor said that he would always have a problem and would not be able to participate in sports.

I saw Roger weekly for two years. I worked a lot with his dural tube, the membrane surrounding the head and the spinal cord, to free it from restrictions, especially at the base of the skull. Rocking it helped to relax him, as did modified still points. I also integrated some Feldenkrais® exercises for the hip, which his mother was very good about doing with him.

Along with this hands-on work, I knew that fundamental changes would also require Roger's "being" to be involved in the process. I tried to engage his imagination to come up with some force that would do the healing on an on-going basis. (For this to be effective the therapist needs to find something that the person can relate to.) Roger's mother said he was into ninjas, so I asked him to imagine some ninjas working in his hip to fix it and make the ball of the femur fit into the joint as it should. He seemed uninterested, and I felt a little discouraged thinking that we would have to try another approach.

The next week when I saw Roger, the first thing he said was that the ninjas were not working in there. The mere mention of this indicated that it was on his mind. I ascertained that the ninjas were indeed in there working away.

As time passed, Roger became interested in sports. He became very good at basketball and baseball. He also loved surfing and skateboarding. His mother was concerned that he might overdo it. I told

---

*Name changed to protect client confidentiality

Roger to let his body be his guide. If anything hurt, he should get a check-up. All continued well.

The doctors were surprised at Roger's progress. They announced that he must have grown out of the problem, as he indeed had—with a little help from some CranioSacral Therapy ninjas.

Aria Rose, MA, CMT, CST
Mill Valley, California
CranioSacral Therapy Practitioner since 1986

Remedy the Cause to Remove the Symptoms

❀ I had recently returned from my second CranioSacral Therapy (CST) seminar and was explaining what I had learned to Barbara,★ a physical therapy assistant with the public school system. She was familiar with my work with children and wanted to know how CST could help her grandson, who was autistic and hyperactive. She immediately asked me to use the CranioSacral techniques on him.

I had the child lie on the floor in a supine position. I started with the CV-4 technique. He demonstrated more flexion tone and began to turn over into the prone fetal position with his face turned to the side and cheek on the floor.

Barbara and I looked at each other and said, "Birth position!" He held this position for about five minutes.

I asked Barbara if the child had experienced any birth trauma. She said labor had been long and that he had been born lifeless and cyanotic. We told him we wanted him to come into the world and that we were happy he was here.

The boy then slowly rose from the floor and went over to a table where there were toys, and he started to quietly play. Barbara let me know that he had never played quietly before.

One of my contracts is with the early intervention service in my state. Through this program I not only work with children, but also teach their parents, parent assistants, teachers, and other caretakers.

Kate was a parent assistant who worked with me in this service. She had seen my work with Down's syndrome children and was concerned about her own baby's progress. Her baby girl was not able to come to a sitting position on her own and was past the

---

★Name changed to protect client confidentiality

age by which this milestone should have been accomplished independently.

Kate asked if I would see her child. Together we agreed on some common goals: to be guided by intuition, to let energy and love perform their work on the baby, and to remain calm through whatever happened.

I performed CranioSacral Therapy with the baby in the supine position. During the CV-4 technique, the baby became very agitated. She raised her left arm above her head and began making a crying/yelping sound. (Interestingly, Kate had had a difficult labor and thinks the baby's arm came out first.)

Kate and I continued to remain calm, telling the baby, "We love you. It's okay to come out. We can't wait to see you."

The baby stopped the yelping. She calmed down. Her body relaxed. And the breathing became slow and deep. She rolled over and looked at her mother.

I gave them an exercise program for developmental skills and made a follow-up appointment for a month later.

In one month they both returned. The baby was not only able to come to a sitting position independently, but she was crawling and pulling herself up to a standing position. She caught up on her milestones and was beginning to pass her peers in skill levels.

CranioSacral Therapy can remedy the cause, which will remove the symptoms.

Karen Pryor, MS, PT
McMinnville, Tennessee
CranioSacral Therapy Practitioner since 2003

A Child Shows the Way

The first time I saw Donnie,* he presented with hypertonicity in the right upper and lower extremities in an extension pattern. He was two years old. He had been diagnosed at the age of twelve months with right-sided spastic cerebral palsy, after showing developmental delays in areas such as crawling and standing.

CranioSacral Therapy (CST) evaluation found his cranial rhythm to be compressed and skewed to the right side, apparently drawn to the right inferior leaf of the tentorium cerebella at the confluence of sinuses.

Because he lacked reciprocal movement, Donnie crawled in a scooting action. When standing or being assisted with walking, he scissored right over left, inverting his ankles and internally rotating at the hips. Any ambulation was with a full assist that included manual placement of the feet in a step-through pattern. His right upper extremity demonstrated weakness, tightness, and some disassociation. He could support a cup or toss a ball only with his left hand.

I saw Donnie on a schedule of two to four times a month. After six months, a number of interesting results were elicited. On several occasions he made a "rebirthing" motion off the side of the table into his mother's arms or lap.

Mouthwork was not readily accepted at first, possibly due to several episodes of tubular feeding in early infancy. Recent work, however, on the vomer and maxilla have led to some dramatic emotional releases and subsequent improvements in verbal skills. In addition to these findings, CST has improved Donnie's appetite (he has gained three to four pounds), decreased tension patterns in his neck and spine by greater than fifty percent, and noticeably improved the body temperature of his hands and feet.

*Name changed to protect client confidentiality

Once-weekly CST sessions are planned with continued monitoring of objective signs.

Richard G. Hofner, MS, PT, ATC, CST
Hamburg, New York
CranioSacral Therapy Practitioner since 1994

Giovanni—A Gift from God

❀ Giovanni was referred to me by a holistic healthcare practitioner who knew that I had recently begun incorporating CranioSacral Therapy into my pediatric occupational therapy practice. His initial visit with me was at the age of three years, nine months, for evaluation and treatment of Pfeiffer's syndrome, consisting of craniosynostosis and aggressive behavior.

A twin born at thirty-two weeks' gestation, Giovanni had a significant birth history. He was removed from his natural mother at the age of two months due to medical neglect. He had severe respiratory problems for his first two years that required a tracheotomy, which further delayed his physical and mental development. Testing at age two years, five months, placed his mental developmental index at seventy-seven, within the mildly delayed range. His behavior was described as highly disorganized, showing signs of hyperactivity, impulsiveness, tantrums, and aggressive behavior. He required constant management by his foster mother (soon to be his adoptive mother) and a private-duty nurse.

When I first met Giovanni and his newly adopted parents, I noted that he was a fragile-appearing little boy with a distorted head and dysmorphic features, which are associated with Pfeiffer's syndrome. In addition, my evaluation revealed sensory deficits that included tactile defensiveness (hypersensitivity to touch) and poor vestibular processing. The vestibular system responds to sensations of movement and affects such diverse functions as muscle tone, balance, visual-motor skills, and attention. He began treatment at the rate of thirty minutes per week.

Although I was eager to get my hands on Giovanni's head, his sensitivity to touch made it very difficult during his early sessions. He was extremely aversive to touch and reacted with fight-or-flight behaviors when I attempted to touch him. My colleagues referred to him as a whirling dervish.

Gradually I was able to place my hands on Giovanni's head and begin to use CranioSacral Therapy techniques. He had a severe override of the parietal bones and the frontal bone, which caused an oddly "pointed" head. The back of his head (occiput) was stuck in place like a shelf over the back of his neck. His cranial rhythm was thready and disorganized. As I monitored his rhythm, I began to sense a softening of the bony restrictions. Over time, there was a gradual separation of the cranial bones.

I have been seeing Giovanni weekly for three years now. Over the course of his treatment, his head has completely remolded. His buzz haircut reveals a normal-looking, symmetrical head. He has had surgery on both of his eyes to allow them to open more fully. In addition to the changes in his physical features, he has shown dramatic progress in his physical and mental development.

Once labeled a "failure to thrive," Giovanni is now tall and well-nourished for his age. Despite his initial low scores in mental development, he is now excelling academically. While his impulsive and occasionally aggressive behaviors have improved, behavior continues to be a problem for him. It is hoped that these issues will resolve further with continued treatment and possibly medication.

My favorite story about Giovanni (and there are many) is that his adoptive parents originally planned to rename him Evan and keep his birth name as a middle name. They changed their minds, however, when they checked the meaning of Giovanni and found that it means "a gift from God."

Lynne Tupper, MPH, OTR, CST
Houston, Texas
CranioSacral Therapy Practitioner since 1998

Born-Again Baby

✿ As a pediatric occupational therapist, I often treat children who have developmental delays. Taylor first came to see me when he was four years old. Diagnosed with autism, he was virtually nonverbal, showed poor eye contact, and had difficulty interacting with his physical and social environment. Since Taylor's symptoms did not become apparent until he was about two and a half years old, his parents had already had his younger brother, Stanton, and Mom was pregnant with sister Annalisa.

Mom and Dad were very vigilant in watching their other children for signs of deficits similar to Taylor's. Even though they had wanted a big family and were wonderful parents, they decided that they wouldn't have more children.

Over the next few years, Taylor progressed very well with the help of Sensory Integration (SI) techniques to calm and organize his disorganized nervous system. During that time I began to explore the benefits of CranioSacral Therapy (CST) with my clients. I took the courses required for pediatric CST and eventually became certified in CST techniques.

Taylor was one of the first children with whom I combined CST and SI techniques. His gains were remarkable. He became a fluent talker; he acquired skills in reading and math; and he gained sufficient social skills to participate in children's choir and tae kwon do. While he continues to have autistic traits, he is well on his way to a happy and productive life.

Despite the parents' resolve to limit the size of their family to three children, they found that number four was on his way. They faced their fourth delivery with both joyful anticipation and concern for the health of their baby. The pregnancy went well, and the whole family looked forward to the new addition.

Unfortunately, the delivery was very difficult for both Baby and Mother. The baby presented feet first and had the cord wrapped around his neck twice. The placenta had separated from the wall of the uterus, causing excessive bleeding. The attending physician determined that an emergency C-section was the only hope to save the baby's life. After several minutes, the baby was delivered.

New son Cavanaugh was whisked off to the neonatal intensive care unit. Estimating that Cavanaugh was one month premature, doctors expressed concern for his health and future development.

I felt both honored and apprehensive when the family asked me to see Cavanaugh for a CST evaluation and treatment. He was one month old by then and weighed five pounds. His color was mottled, his breathing shallow, and he was curled up like a ball. He lay on Dad's shoulder, so tiny and curled up that his spine showed through his thin skin, like a ridge down the middle of his back. His muscles were so tense that he was difficult to hold. He was too weak to cry. His suck was so poor that he could not nurse.

Dad carried Cavanaugh into a treatment room and placed him on his tummy on a platform swing. He rocked the swing gently, and I carefully turned Cavanaugh onto his back to begin his first CST session. Initiating the protocol I had learned for infants, I placed my hands on his chest and abdomen to release his respiratory diaphragm. Almost immediately he took in a big breath. His breathing moved from his upper chest to his tummy, and his color turned to pink. I placed a finger under his neck and rolled his head back, cradling it in my hands. I gently held this position to evaluate for movement and symmetry, and to allow any restrictions to self-correct. His cranial rhythm was barely apparent; it felt thready and irregular. It moved slowly and had a restricted range of motion.

As I held Cavanaugh's head in my hands, the rhythm increased slowly and became stronger and more regular. I placed my pinky finger in his mouth to free up any restrictions in the soft palate. He began to suck my finger with greater force. I continued the evaluation by gently working at the sacrum. I felt a gentle relaxation of the tension in the dural tube. He seemed fragile and fatigued, so I turned him on his tummy to rest.

I thought the session had gone well and was satisfied to stop before he became too tired. He, on the other hand, had another agenda entirely. As he lay on the swing, he began to push himself toward me with his feet and legs. He was approaching the edge of the swing when his mom and I realized that he was assuming the proper position for delivery. Having observed an instructor use his body to form a cervix for a child, I cupped my hands into a circle about three or four inches in diameter.

Cavanaugh continued to kick and push his head into and then through my hands. His head went down and through and then up again as it emerged from my hands. His body lengthened and stretched out. I moved my hands to catch him as he pushed off the edge of the swing. I placed him back on the swing on his tummy. He took another deep breath and let out a cry for his mother, who fed him a two-ounce bottle of milk. We laughed at the thought of a born-again baby.

When we took Cavanaugh back to the waiting room, Dad commented that he was easier to hold because he was relaxed and could stretch out on his shoulder. Since that day, his breathing and suck have continued to improve, and he has begun to nurse.

A month after Cavanaugh's first treatment, he met his developmental milestones as an alert and interactive infant. He has recently been diagnosed with trisomy-21 (Down's syndrome). We have no idea how his future development will progress. However, we plan to follow him with both standardized testing and clinical observations.

Cavanaugh's parents credit CST with his progress to date. They plan to continue regular CST and are hopeful that he will continue to make developmental gains. Cavanaugh is a miracle baby and a blessing to us all.

Lynne Tupper, MPH, OTR, CST
Houston, Texas
CranioSacral Therapy Practitioner since 1998

Opening the Lines of Communication

✿ One of my clients brought her seven-year-old granddaughter Makayla to my office. Makayla did not speak more than two or three words at a time, did not read well, and was having difficulty in school.

Her cranium felt very compressed, mostly in the parietals and the saggital suture. Her rhythm was very slow, and her head and neck felt compressed down into her shoulders. As she lay on the table and I applied the vault holds, her mother and grandmother sat at the side of the office and whispered. Her mother thought something had happened to Makayla at a relative's house. Just as she made this statement, Makayla's body started to vibrate, and I sensed that her mother had verbalized what Makayla's body was trying to communicate.

Makayla went into a deeper significant state and started to release from the top of her head. Her cranial bones started to make major shifts, and the reduction in pressure could be felt. Her body felt more relaxed, and so I proceeded to apply the individual cranial bone releases, followed by the dural rock and glide. Her dural tube stretched and felt like it took a deep breath.

By the end of the session Makayla's eyes looked more alert, and she appeared more relaxed than when she first arrived. She got off the table and went to her grandmother and thanked her for bringing her there. All three left the office feeling happy with their decision to bring Makayla for a session.

Afterward I learned that Makayla was asked a question at the dinner table and, instead of responding with her usual two or three words, answered in a complete sentence. Everyone was taken by surprise. After that, Makayla spoke complete sentences and became a bit of a "Chatty Cathy"—probably trying to make up the lost time.

Makayla's whole family was happily surprised by the results from just one session. I encouraged Makayla's mother to continue Cranio-

Sacral Therapy when they returned to their hometown, which they did for a while. Reports are that Makayla's schoolwork has improved wonderfully and she interacts more with family and friends.

Lucy Franqui Gustitis, NCTMB
Kalispell, Montana
CranioSacral Therapy Practitioner since 2000

A Rose Is a Rose

❀ I had been practicing CranioSacral Therapy for ten years when I got the calling to work with babies. I was neither seeking nor expecting the fateful request that came one winter morning from a desperate first-time mother. Her three-week-old daughter Rose had been born prematurely and, although she had been released from the hospital, she could not nurse for more than a few seconds, was startled by every sound, and woke up from every nap screaming.

Rose had been through numerous medical tests, but no physical pathologies were found. Nonetheless, her pediatrician recommended anti-seizure medications. Mom could not stand that idea and felt in her heart that her baby was trying to tell her something. As a last-ditch effort, she called me on the advice of a friend I had helped with headaches months before.

Mother and baby Rose arrived early for our first session looking drawn, exhausted, and terrified. Rose was screaming inconsolably, and Mother was crying and visibly shaken. I asked Mom to let me treat her first to help her relax a bit and know that the work was safe.

On the table, Mom was rigidly holding her chest, and her breath was very rapid and shallow. She said she felt as if life itself was being drained out of her by the stress of caring for her panicked infant and not knowing what to do to help. As I worked to calm and stabilize her nervous system, I realized that both she and her baby were in shock from birth traumas. I explained that our work together would focus on helping both of them release the shock and fear so that they could relax and enjoy each other.

After about thirty minutes of cranial work Mom relaxed and began to breathe deeply. Her shoulders and chest softened and she began to sob softly, explaining how difficult and disappointing the whole birth experience had been for her. As if on cue, Rose stopped crying as her mother told me the sad story. I picked up Rose and brought her to the table to be cradled in Mom's arms. I asked Mom to keep telling the birth story softly as she cuddled her infant, and I encouraged their eye contact.

I invited Rose to show me what she needed help with, as I lightly touched her chest with one hand and supported her back with the other. Immediately her little chest went rigid as she arched backwards and began to scream hysterically. I could feel the terror in her lungs and hear it in her cry. It was heart-rending, and I found myself talking to Rose directly, empathizing with her birth experience and inviting her to let go of her pain and fear now that Mom and I were there to help her. Rose continued to scream and cough but was present in her eyes, as if holding onto us as she experienced the storm in her body. As we worked, the screams changed to crying, and she finally softened and relaxed her body.

After resting a few minutes, Rose tried to nurse but soon became agitated and started screaming again. With Mom's permission I gently worked to synchronize the baby's suck reflex with her cranial rhythm until she was strong in the suck reflex on my finger. Much to our delight, Rose then returned to the breast for a successful feeding. We were all exhausted, but much had been learned and we were all encouraged.

I asked Mom and Baby to return weekly for the next six weeks. At each session I helped Mom renegotiate her fear during her daughter's birth and neonatal period, delving into her own birth trauma and exploring how that was expressed in her birthing experience. As she worked through her own fear she became more calm and confident as a mother. Her calmness reassured Rose, and they began a healthy bonding process.

Each session I worked with the baby to release tensions held in the chest and throat and to maintain a vital suck reflex. I also did a few sessions with Dad to ease his anxiety.

Soon Rose was crying less frequently, feeding better, and gaining weight. By the end of the sixth session Rose was sleeping through the night and feeding normally at the breast. Home life had become manageable, even pleasurable! Mother and Baby continued to come for sessions once a month for about six months, and then as needed when illness or injury would trigger Rose back into screaming.

Rose, her parents, and I have all become good friends in the three years since we first came together for healing that winter evening. Mom is calm and happy and is considering how she wants her next pregnancy and birth to be. Rose is a happy, curious, drug-free, active toddler enjoying her life and family. Dad is at ease in his life knowing that his wife and daughter are well and happy.

Since baby Rose came to show me how easy it can be to work with infants, I have taken training in pediatric CranioSacral Therapy and am now treating babies regularly. My tiny clients continue to show me how to help them. There is an incredible opportunity present at birth to become aware of how a safe, gentle, bonded birth experience supports love and trust, and how even a violent birth experience can be renegotiated.

What we give always comes back to bless us. And so it was for me with baby Rose, who came to initiate my work with babies and pointed me in the direction of my next career path: learning how to create nonviolent birth experiences for families of the future.

Ellen Costantino, CST
Caledonia, Michigan
CranioSacral Therapy Practitioner since 1996

Infant Relieved of Respiratory Distress

❀ When I first met Johnny, he was a six-month-old infant. As he rested comfortably in his mother's arms, she explained to me that he had already been hospitalized four times for respiratory infections and had been diagnosed with bronchiectasis. Pregnancy and childbirth had been uneventful, and there was no apparent reason for his frequent infections.

Johnny appeared to be satisfied and healthy that day, but his breathing was somewhat shallow, not the full, deep breathing that we usually observe in infants. I placed one hand on the lower ribs and upper belly, and the other slightly lower on his back, as his mother continued to hold him. Soon he began crying loudly and vigorously.

Mom reached for the bottle with her free hand. "No, don't," I said. "He needs to cry. See how his lungs are opening up. See how deeply he is breathing. He needs this."

She stopped but appeared quite uncomfortable and distressed as I held his diaphragm and he bawled.

After about fifteen or twenty minutes, the crying subsided and I removed my hands. Johnny snuggled into his mother's arms. He turned to look at me with a huge grin on his face, his small eyes brimming with love and joy. "I think I'm forgiven," I said to Mom, seeking to reassure her that her child had not been traumatized.

I had two more sessions with Johnny during which I worked with his diaphragm as well as his cranium. Both times, he relaxed and appeared content, with no further crying. The frequent respiratory infections ceased, and there were no further hospitalizations.

Johnny's experience was what we refer to as SomatoEmotional Release.® He cried not because I injured or frightened him, but because he was releasing pent-up emotion that he had stored physically. The stored emotion was preventing him from breathing freely, and he was subject to frequent respiratory infections. After his emotions were released and breathing became free, he was able to resist infections and be a normal, healthy child.

I have not seen Johnny for several years now, but I have spoken with his grandmother. She assures me that he has remained healthy and has needed no further hospitalization.

Ann Harman, DO
Micanopy, Florida
CranioSacral Therapy Practitioner since 1986

CST to the Sleep Rescue

❀ My three-year-old grandson Michael was spending the night with us. He is a very active and over-imaginative little guy. He has great manners, but because of a traumatic birth he is edgy, has insomnia, and exhibits other nervous system overactivity.

After we laid him down for the night, he ventured back into our room crying four different times, using every excuse under the sun as to why he was unable to fall asleep. First he saw shadows. Then he heard noises. Then he was thirsty.

An insomniac from birth, Michael kept saying, "I don't know how to sleep." We tried comforting him in a number of ways. We read stories. We created a quiet atmosphere. We explained that when you relax, sleep just comes. Finally, we just gave in and resorted to saying, "Go to sleep!" By now it was two a.m. and I was very tired. (This was one of the reasons we had him for the night—to give his parents some sleep time.) I told my husband, "I think I can at least get him relaxed."

I gently decompressed Michael's thoracic inlet and began some CranioSacral Therapy (CST). Immediately he began to twitch, and I felt the cerebrospinal fluid filling around the sutures. Within less than two minutes, he was breathing heavily, his body was limp and fully relaxed, and he was sound asleep! My husband declared it a miracle.

Michael didn't even wake up when we moved him. He slept soundly all night. In fact, he actually slept two hours longer than he normally did at home—all from just one CST mini session!

Now my daughter brings Michael to me for regular appointments. His nervous system is showing a definite improvement on a daily basis. She also notices that his appetite has improved and his allergies are minimal.

Karen S. McGill, ND
New Buffalo, Michigan
CranioSacral Therapy Practitioner since 2003

Simply Stated, Yet Profound

❀ Being a mom who is also a CranioSacral Therapy (CST) provider, I've often wondered (and privately feared) what effect the complicated pregnancy I went through had on my son Jacob *in utero*.

I had a rare condition known as vasoprevia during my pregnancy. The cord was completely embedded into the membranes of the sac and crossed the cervix, leaving very little free-flowing cord. In addition, the cord had only two vessels instead of the normal three, which meant that Jacob wasn't receiving the normal amount of nutrients.

We learned from the doctors that if Jacob dropped in position, or if my water broke and I went into labor, we would lose him because his blood supply would be cut off.

We had no choice but to schedule a C-section. Not only did Jacob have to be delivered this way, he was positioned so high up that suction was also utilized during the delivery. Had he been positioned lower, however, he would have been compressing his own blood supply.

The C-section with suction combination is a nightmare to a CranioSacral Therapist, but this occurred before I embarked on the CST journey. Based on what I know now, I believe this played into Jacob's other problems, which included difficulty latching on, profuse spitting up, and numerous ear infections.

Jacob is now three and has received several CranioSacral Therapy treatments. In December 2003 I had the pleasure of attending a class on pediatric applications of CST at The Upledger Institute HealthPlex clinic. I was fortunate to be able to bring Jacob, thanks to a friend who accompanied me to babysit.

While we were there, Jacob received a profound treatment. He bonded well with one of the therapists, who really tuned into his umbilicus region. Following the treatment, Jacob—then just two months shy of age three—looked up directly into my eyes and without being prompted said, "He sucked my boo-boo out." This was then followed by "I liked being in your belly."

Shannon Desilets, PT
Pembroke, New Hampshire
CranioSacral Therapy Practitioner since 2002

Twin Catches Up

✿ A client became the proud grandmother of twin girls, Mary and Emma, who appeared normal at birth. By their first birthday, however, a number of developmental and behavioral differences had become apparent.

Emma, the second born, had been delivered hastily with forceps while under fetal distress. She displayed excessive thumb sucking, head banging, irritability, and frequent crying for no obvious reason. Developmentally, she crawled and walked later than normal, had poorer eye-hand coordination, and showed difficulty focusing and paying attention.

Emma's parents brought her in at eighteen months of age for a CranioSacral Therapy session. Mom's intuition told her that it would help Emma. Dad was wary of anything not prescribed by the twins' pediatrician, but he attended the session to see what would happen.

After spending a short time talking to the parents and helping Emma settle down, we found it best for Dad to hold the squirming child while another therapist used blowing soap bubbles as a distraction.

Upon checking Emma's craniosacral rhythm, I found only the rate to be normal. Her symmetry was out of phase in flexion and extension. The amplitude was restricted on both sides, with the right being the least open. In addition, the rhythm demonstrated the qualities of low energy and a weakened vitality with a rough motion.

The extent of these imbalances required the entire 10-Step Protocol, plus unwinding for a complete treatment. Even though unwinding is often accomplished early on in a toddler session, Emma didn't respond until after the full 10-Step was finished and unwinding was repeated. During the session she became noticeably more relaxed, with rosier cheeks. All qualities improved, especially her energy and vitality.

Several months later, her grandmother reported that Emma had stopped banging her head and rarely sucked her thumb or cried. Developmentally and behaviorally she had become much like her fraternal twin Mary.

It was rewarding and impressive to see so much improvement after only a single session, especially in recognition of the fact that so great a number of imbalances often requires additional treatments.

Jeanne Girard, MA, CNMT
Canon City, Colorado
CranioSacral Therapy Practitioner since 1988

Scott McGee
Canon City, Colorado
CranioSacral Therapy Practitioner since 1995

Accident's Effects Return to Haunt Teen

❀ As a daring teen, Eric★ tested the limits, until one day they tested him. In 1997, at the age of sixteen, he and a friend crashed their motorcycle into a tree at high speed.

With the miracle of medicine and time, Eric's brain repaired itself and a portion of his crushed frontal right skull was replaced with a metal plate. Some physical injuries healed while others, such as his right eye, did not. After a year in recovery and rehab, his humor and enthusiasm for life reasserted itself. He returned to high school, graduated, and began his career in an automotive shop he co-owned with his father.

Four years later, in 2001, something went wrong. Eric began to lose physical strength and coordination. His consciousness became fuzzy, he lost his balance, his speech deteriorated, and his blood pressure and endocrine system went out of whack. For months the family transported him weekly to the university research hospital for testing. Nothing was working. In a period of six months, he went from being an active, robust young man to being wheelchair-bound in a half-conscious, near-vegetative state. His balance, his mind, his entire system seemed to be shutting down. The state granted him full disability under Social Security, and the hospital sent him home with no hope of further treatment.

Coming from a small town, I had followed Eric's case through mutual friends. News of the recent downturn caused me to reflect on stories I had heard during my various hands-on studies. Because of the trauma history, I suspected that the extreme symptoms might be mitigated with massage methods designed to support cranial balance and scar-tissue release.

Through an acquaintance I offered to work with Eric on an experimental basis, and the family called to accept. The first week we

---

★Name changed to protect patient confidentiality

did short fifteen-minute sessions every other day at his home, letting him remain in the wheelchair. The work was light, a combination of CranioSacral Therapy and myofascial release of scar tissues. He responded from the first session.

The early focus was at the base of the occiput to restore range of motion to the head. Heavy internal scarring had thickened the tissues, effectively freezing the head/neck joint. The impact of the crash had messed with the inner tissues of the skull, brain, and face, leaving the structure out of balance with little or no sacral pulse. Head trauma and injury had left a web of scarring over the face and skull.

We worked together well, and the results were profound and immediately evident. In two weeks, Eric was able to stand and stay awake more. We moved him to the bed, which allowed me better access to the whole body, especially the sacrum. By four weeks the heavy slurring in his speech was changing. Once he began to see the progress, his motivation kicked in. By six weeks he was moving. He soon walked the driveway without help.

Over the next two months Eric took matters to their logical conclusion: He began running. Before long he had regained his balance. His speech became clear. He rebalanced his left/right symmetry. He returned to work. He began driving to my office for his sessions. And he joined the health club. Every few months we do one or two sessions to fine-tune and maintain.

It is a privilege to build a relationship with a client. It is a joy to watch a transformation. But, more than anything, it is a gift to be given the tools to make a difference.

Lesley Waldron, LMT
CranioSacral Therapy Practitioner since 1999
Location withheld to protect patient confidentiality

Witnessing a Miracle

Two years ago a beautiful four-year-old autistic boy came to see me with his mom. He didn't make eye contact, didn't seem to have speech, and when I tried to put him on my treatment table he strongly resisted.

For the first seven sessions I worked the best I could to free his severely bound cranial mechanism. He was difficult to work on, as he screamed at the top of his lungs for the entire forty-five-minute session. The screaming would begin the moment he got on my table and end as soon as I finished.

The boy would thrash around and twist his head in every direction trying to get away, as I did my best to hold on and try to enhance his cranial rhythm. He also used his hands to push my fingers off his head. I got kicked in the head more than once as I was working. His mom must have had tremendous faith to go through all that screaming with her child. She was extremely helpful and did her best to hold her son as I worked on him.

Each session we would get some releases, but nothing dramatic. His head was still very tight, and there seemed to be little force at the center of his craniosacral system to try and break free.

Then came the miraculous eighth session. It began as usual with the screaming, twisting, and trying to get away from my firm, yet gentle, hands. During the work I would pray that I was being respectful to this child's soul, as he was being forced against his will each week for forty-five minutes.

I was solidly holding an energy cyst that was right at the center of his craniosacral mechanism. All of a sudden, like magic, he stopped screaming and fell deeply asleep as this cyst released. He began to release and twitch all over. He had one release after another. His cranial rhythm was tremendously improved.

This beautiful boy was deep asleep for the next twenty minutes until the session ended. We let him sleep a little bit more, but I needed to get him up, as there was another client waiting.

When he got up he looked me straight in the eye and said, "Mr. Jokel, I want to hug you." He was soft and warm and loving.

I was very excited on my way home that day, believing that I just witnessed a miracle. When next week came around, I feared that he would have reverted to his previous way of being, but he was still greatly improved.

We continued to work together over the next two years, and I now see him about every six weeks. He is, for all intents and purposes, a normal six-year-old child. He makes eye contact, has long conversations, does well in all his subjects in school, and relates well to other children and adults. He is very easy to love, and is very loving in return.

Robert Jokel, PT
Mahopac, New York
CranioSacral Therapy Practitioner since 1986

Showing Where It Hurts

A mother brought in her eighteen-month-old son Justin* to see me. He suffered from winter colds and ear infections, and he was easily irritated. She mentioned that he occasionally hit his head against the wall.

Upon palpation, I found a depression on the right side of Justin's head, a tightness at the base of the skull, and compressed sphenoid and temporal bones. I was unable to work with him on the table. He would not cooperate and wanted to go to his mother whenever I started to work on him. He was more interested in me reading a story to him or playing with the toys in our office.

In conversation I mentioned to Justin's mother that even little babies will sometimes take my hand and put it where they need help. At that moment Justin grabbed my hand and stuck it in his mouth while he was being held by his mother. There was no resistance except for closing of the mouth on my finger.

I propped open his mouth with my other hand and went straight for the vomer, the bone that joins the two halves of the maxilla or upper jaw. It was jammed into the palatine complex and further up into the sphenoid. I held the sphenoid and maxilla and decompressed the vomer from the spheno-palatine complex. I felt it float down as it released.

Justin immediately fell asleep. The mother was perplexed. I explained that when something releases, it is a relief and the body relaxes, sometimes to the point of sleep.

We put Justin on the table and I continued to work easily without interference, releasing the sacrum and then the ethmoid bone at the top of the maxilla. He was in a deep sleep and stayed that way for one and a half hours after he left the office.

---

*Name changed to protect client confidentiality

The mother later reported that Justin seemed better, not so irritated and more relaxed. The plans are for him to come in for a follow-up after their summer vacation.

Aria Rose, MA, CMT, CST
Mill Valley, California
CranioSacral Therapy Practitioner since 1986

Marvelous Mac

❁ As his mother let go of his hood, Mac burst into the room and immediately started ripping out the plants in my fountain. Wow! His mother looked at me and said, "This is going to be a very expensive visit." I knew right away from her sense of humor that I was really going to like this woman.

Her son Mac was a six-year-old autistic dynamo. He was quite large for his age and had the most warm, brown, heart-melting eyes. When he spoke I couldn't understand any of the words, unless he was repeating what I had just said; then it was easier to guess. Mac quickly went through all the toys and zeroed in on a writing toy. He may not have been able to speak, but, boy, could he spell!

Mom told me that Mac was very aggressive in school; he would pinch the other children. It was also very hard for him to focus. I noticed that his eyes never looked at me, but just darted around the room.

Working with him was at first a bit challenging. His mom was wonderful. She would hold on to him or just support him. It was a bit of "catch me if you can"—and I did! I am used to working in the world of pediatrics on the run. I have to say, though, in the beginning Mac wasn't happy.

I started by seeing him once a week; then I saw him every other week. As the treatments progressed, I was able to meld and blend more and more. His behavior responded to this, and he became calmer. As the membranes began to move, I think Mac decided that this wasn't too bad. His behavior at school was improving, and the pinching had lessened. As time went on, he became calmer and more settled.

The real breakthrough in his speech started after he received mouth work. I had finally reached a point where I thought I could trust him enough to not bite. There were a few close calls, but we both knew that this was making a difference. Mac's vomer was up so high and was very compressed. His maxilla had very little movement. What a difference it made to have mobility restored in those facial bones. Now, Mac not only takes mouth work in stride, he moves my finger or fingers to where he needs the release.

I will never forget what happened on one occasion after the mouth work was completed for the day. As I withdrew my gloved finger from his mouth, he said at least four sentences in what sounded like perfect Japanese. I looked at his mother, and we were both wide-eyed. Feeling completely surprised, I said to his mother, "Oh, that's right, you wanted him to speak English!" We both laughed, but he never ceases to amaze me.

Mac has taught me so much. One day he took his hand and put my finger back into his mouth. He has taught me to make sure that *he* is finished with the release, because he's the one who really knows how to heal himself. His mom has commented that she can tell when he is really in a good spot (a release) because his feet move.

I have been seeing Mac for almost four years now. His aggression has stopped. He makes great eye contact. And his speaking ability is greatly improved; in fact, it is a rare occasion that I cannot understand what he says. His teachers and aides are amazed at his progress.

When I haven't seen Mac for a while, or he goes through a growth spurt and the membranes get tighter, he has been known to cut his hair in just the area that needs some release. His mom keeps an eye out for that—and the scissors hidden!

One night, several months ago, Mac woke up crying. He went to his mom and dad's bedside at two in the morning. Remembering how well her son was now communicating, she asked him what was wrong. He said, "Ear hurt." She was in tears when she told me how much that meant to her. I think that says it all.

Donna L. Busse, RRT, LMT, NCTMB, CST-D
Cincinnati, Ohio
CranioSacral Therapy Practitioner since 1996

The Real Face of Gabriel

✤ Little Gabriel was my last patient of the day. His parents had learned about CranioSacral Therapy through their desperate search for help for their new baby.

Since his birth, Gabriel had grown some in length but had lost more than a pound of weight. Projectile vomiting along with difficulty swallowing were prohibiting him from receiving the nourishment he needed to put on the pounds.

Gabriel still looked much like a newborn, though longer and very stressed. His eyes were bulging out, which gave him a look of being constantly frightened or being squeezed too tightly. He was scared, frustrated, hungry and, at first, could not relax his body while in my arms.

For our first half hour together, Gabriel continued with his usual forceful vomiting pattern. He had no awareness of nor interest in his environment. He was lost in his agony and didn't even have the strength to cry.

According to his parents, Gabriel's birth had been beautiful. Mom's labor was short, easy, and unmedicated, and Gabriel entered the world in calm surroundings. Mother and baby spent the first hour post-delivery getting acquainted with each other. By medical standards, Gabriel's arrival was textbook-perfect.

Yet this newborn was struggling to a degree that made me wonder if he should be in a hospital. Was there more to this than what I could see? Just then his little body finally began to relax in my hands. From that point on Gabriel gave himself over to the therapy with total trust. In fact, he seemed to take over. His little face showed serious concentration, as if he knew exactly what was happening. He followed every move, every change with serious intensity.

Gabriel's body guided my hands so expertly that there was no question in my mind he knew where he was going. He only needed my hands to follow. I had no doubt that this tiny being possessed understanding of the wisdom of his cells, and he wasted no time. He was making use of all he could get from this session. He never lost concentration, and he did not vacillate. He was like the little train that just kept going.

For Gabriel's parents it was a relief to see him so relaxed. Watching the session itself, though, must have been like watching grass grow. A light touch here. A different hand position there. Hold here. Touch there. Yet they observed with great interest, noticing Gabriel's every breath, every little movement, every change. They commented periodically on the differences they were seeing: how his facial expression was changing, how he no longer had the frightened look, how his mouth opened so wide as he yawned.

It was at this point that I picked up on the interaction between Gabriel and each of his parents. The three of them had a silent way of communicating that incredibly they all understood. It was like a circle encompassing all of them. Gabriel's mother was still guiding this child, just as she had done during the birth process.

I invited both Mother and Father to place a hand on their baby. Gabriel sighed and then began to cry as if he were telling a sad story. When he was finished he lay in my arms, looking like a different child. His little face relaxed, his eyes were no longer bulging, and the vomiting had stopped.

More than two hours had passed since we started the session. Now, for the first time since Gabriel's birth eight weeks prior, his parents were seeing the real face of their son.

Ilona E. Trommler, LMT
Westlake, Ohio
CranioSacral Therapy Practitioner since 1998

Case of Mystery Seizures Solved

About a year ago, a mother brought her two-and-a-half-year-old son to me to be evaluated. He had had seven epileptic-like seizures in the previous month—almost two per week.

The concerned parents had taken their son to specialists, but tests found no cause for these terrible seizures. The last seizure, worse than the previous ones, had resulted in the boy losing control of his bladder functions. The only recommendation was to put the child on anti-seizure medication. The parents did not want to do this.

In town from Georgia, the couple asked a relative for someone in the alternative field who might help their son. They were told to call me and see what I could do.

An evaluation of the sphenoid bone movement showed a strong side-bending motion. I worked to correct this imbalance. This was very difficult to do on a young child who did not want to stay still. What worked was for the mother to lie on the table and put the child face down on her stomach. In an hour of time we probably got in about fifteen minutes of actual movement therapy. Working on him during his regular nap time helped, since he went to sleep. Though I had just three days to work with him, it was apparently enough to stop the seizures.

This was a child who had not experienced any big falls. His birth had not been difficult. There had been no forceps or suction delivery. There was no obvious reason for an incident of this severity to occur. What worked was plain CranioSacral Therapy.

Since this family lived near Atlanta, I gave them the numbers for The Upledger Institute HealthPlex clinic and urged the parents to take the boy there for an evaluation. Able to locate a therapist near their home, they sought treatment there. The last I heard, the boy was doing fine.

Park Bishop, LMT
Richardson, Texas
CranioSacral Therapy Practitioner since 1999

CST Supports a Pregnancy

❀ A few years ago, J.W., a young mother of two, came into my office for massage therapy for injuries she had received in a car accident. About a year after her final appointment, she returned stressed and depressed about a recent miscarriage. She had a few massage appointments and then disappeared again. Soon she was back—another miscarriage. Then another.

I finally suggested that we try CranioSacral Therapy (CST). We would work with whatever part of the body seemed to be needing attention at the time of treatment. She loved it. She said she felt even better than after a massage, and her body responded beautifully to the light-touch therapy.

After several sessions of CST over a few months, she announced that she was pregnant again. This time, I suggested she come in every couple of weeks to see if we could do something to help her body support this pregnancy.

As the weeks went by, I worked on the baby and her mom together, assisting with their relationship and exchange of fluids, nutrients, oxygen, and so on.

At term, J.W. had a scheduled C-section. I arrived at the hospital shortly after delivery to work on the newborn. The baby was beautiful, but very asymmetrical in her cranium. One side of her mouth was turned up, the other side down. One eye was open, the other closed. One ear was sticking out, the other was flat.

As I talked with Mom, I held the baby in my lap, her feet to my chest and her occiput resting in the palms of my cupped hands. I suddenly felt the occiput shifting in my hands. It felt like a bag of worms. Within a minute, the shifting subsided. I looked down and she was perfectly symmetrical! The proud parents saw the marked difference and were even prouder.

Today, this beautiful girl is almost three, and her parents proclaim she continues to be the best baby ever—extremely healthy, alert, inquisitive, a great sleeper, and never cries except when truly necessary.

Recently, in a note of thanks, Mom and Dad credited Cranio-Sacral Therapy for helping to maintain and nurture the pregnancy, for bringing a healthy little girl into the world, and for giving them the least problematic child on the planet.

Barbara Nelen, LMT
Winter Park, Florida
CranioSacral Therapy Practitioner since 1997

Search for Help Crosses Continents

✺ Rafael is a seven-year-old boy from Africa diagnosed with severe autism. His family moved to the United States in order to find better services for him. He scored fifty-seven initially on the Childhood Autism Rating Scale, which is the highest end of the severely autistic range.

Rafael was essentially nonverbal, very aggressive, and scared of people. He experienced nightly sleep disturbances. He was highly agitated and difficult to console, which are traits of social and language disabilities within the autism spectrum. Severe motor disturbances (executional praxis) were also apparent, as he could not imitate any actions or carry out independent motions.

Rafael was referred to our clinic for occupational therapy with Sensory Integration, but the family was seeking CranioSacral Therapy as well. He was enrolled in a private special education program and received speech therapy at another clinic.

Though the entire craniosacral system first appeared to be completely restricted, there was eventually a cranial rhythm detected in the feet. Still point inductions were the primary means of intervention for several weeks.

A significant finding was compression at the anterior-posterior cranial base. The dural tube was pulled tightly three-dimensionally and was most easily worked on from the sacral region. Cranial sutures were not only tight and immobile, but touch to each suture was very painful to this child at first. Slow and gentle intrusion into his system was the pace. The 10-Step Protocol for pediatrics was the guideline for intervention. The parietal lift technique was a consistent method that seemed to bring on many behavioral improvements.

CranioSacral Therapy was the primary treatment for at least four months and then was often halted for several weeks, either due to scheduling conflicts or by choice to test its effectiveness. There were consistent recurrences of behavioral deterioration during each of the pauses in treatment.

By the six-month mark, eighty percent of Rafael's intervention was CranioSacral Therapy. By this time he was sleeping through each night, plus the family found it quite easy to direct him toward bed. They used to have to drive him around for miles to help him fall asleep every night. This had been their ritual for nine years of their son's life.

Rafael began to follow simple directions and to use four or five signs for communication. He was also starting to utter recognizable words at times. This improvement did not emerge until the onset of CranioSacral Therapy, even though he had received work in this area for months prior.

Another change was in Rafael's behavior at school. The day used to consist of the staff preventing him from hurting himself or others. Now he was able to participate in the learning process. His aggression, manifested in grabbing people by the throat, had been reduced by ninety to ninety-five percent. (He would still resort to this communication tactic during extreme moments of stress.)

There was significant increase in eye contact, smiling, and overall mood improvement. Rafael showed agitation less than ten percent of the time. Eventually it became clear that an underlying illness was imminent at these times of behavioral deteriorations. During the six months prior to the start of CranioSacral Therapy, he used to cry incessantly. Crying was now reported as being minimal, even rare, occurring only when he was not feeling well. This improvement was a major relief for his parents and other family members.

Rafael's father, who is a scientist, especially wanted the CranioSacral Therapy to continue as part of his son's ongoing health management.

Susan Vaughan Kratz, OTR, BCP
Waukesha, Wisconsin
CranioSacral Therapy Practitioner since 2000

Jackie Kucharski, OTR
Cedarburg, Wisconsin
CranioSacral Therapy Practitioner since 2002

Anna's Pot of Gold at the End of the Rainbow

❁ I am a massage therapist and bodyworker for a variety of reasons. One is that I enjoy helping others. Another is that I love getting paid to do what I love. As I discovered with one client, however, the best payment sometimes comes in forms other than money.

Anna★ is a fifteen-year-old girl who lives with her older sister Cherie★ because her relationship with her mother is difficult. Anna and Cherie came in one day to get massages. Anna looked like she had a dark cloud hanging over her head. My massage therapist husband worked with Cherie, and I worked with Anna.

Anna had never had a massage before. We began by discussing her history. She had some low back pain and tension, plus she experienced constant headaches, migraines, and depression. Anna told me that she had felt depression for as long as she could remember. (Any amount of time is too long for a fifteen-year-old to have depression.) She told me that on two occasions, when she was in first and sixth grades, she had fallen and split open her chin. She also told me that she had injured her tailbone. On top of all that, she had a hard time sleeping.

In listening to her difficulties, I realized that she was one who could benefit from CranioSacral Therapy (CST). I told Anna a bit about the technique. I described what a session was like, and how her accidents in grade school could have contributed to her headaches, migraines, depression, sleep difficulties, and even her low back pain. I told her I understood that she came expecting a "rub my muscles and make me feel good" type of massage, and if that was all she wanted, I would give her that. I let her know, though, that a CST session would be just as relaxing, plus it could be therapeutically very helpful.

★Names changed to protect client confidentiality

It made a lot of sense to Anna that her accidents could have caused these long-term difficulties. She definitely felt that something was "off" or "not right." She wanted to give it a try. She'd try anything to help her situation. She didn't like being in pain and depressed.

We started her off with some time on a Still Point Inducer. Five minutes later, she was smiling—her headache was gone!

I proceeded to do a 10-Step Protocol. During the session my hands worked with a body that was tight. Her sacrum and sphenoid were both very compressed. I was glad we were able to offer her body a time and space to start letting go of the trauma it had sustained and held on to for years. By the end of her session her cranial rhythm was stronger and more full. Anna had even fallen into a deep sleep.

When she came out of the treatment room to meet up with her sister she was glowing! Not knowing what to call her first experience of CranioSacral Therapy, she said, "That was the best back rub ever! I feel like I'm high—a good high!"

The fifteen-year-old who walked into my office that evening under a dark rain cloud walked out with no headache. Best of all, the sparkle in her eyes and the huge smile on her face made her look as if she had found a pot of gold at the end of a rainbow.

Seeing Anna like that was the best payment a client has ever given me. It is very rewarding knowing that I helped Anna, and I have continued to do so, relieving her headaches and depression to the point that she can spend better time at home with Mom.

Julie McKay, CMT, RBFP
Madison, Wisconsin
CranioSacral Therapy Practitioner since 1998

A Headache-Free Christmas

✿ I was introduced to CranioSacral Therapy when my own daughter was treated for recurring ear infections. Seeing how quickly and completely she was cured using this therapy spawned a desire in me to learn it myself. I have used what I learned since then to help so many others.

One of my clients was fifteen-year-old Amy. I first saw her when she came to Florida to spend Christmas with her aunt Mary Jo and family. Mary Jo, a client of mine, called to ask if I would be able to do an immediate treatment on her niece. The only time I had available was Christmas Eve and the day after Christmas. We set up two appointments.

Amy was in a great deal of pain, and had been ever since playing Helen Keller in a school play. Her role had required her to fall a lot. One of the times she fell she hit her head on a chair, which triggered her troubles.

Upon the play's completion, Amy found herself having severe migraine headaches, complete with nausea and sensitivity to light. After Amy spent several days in great discomfort, her parents took her to the emergency room. There she was given medication, which she had an allergic reaction to. She was referred to a neurologist, and her appointment was scheduled for that upcoming January.

When Amy arrived at my home on Christmas Eve, I could tell she was in a lot of pain. While arcing, I immediately found problems in her parietal and upper cervicals. Passing my hands over her body to survey, I found that the parietals were bowed out superiorly along the frontal suture. Along the temporal suture I found that the parietal was pushed in on her left side. I also found that her atlas had been extended posteriorly beyond C2 [cervical vertebra]. I began a complete 10-Step Protocol, while focusing on the area of concern.

Working with the parietal during the 10-Step, it was necessary to use direction of energy as well as the parietal techniques to move the bones back into their correct alignment. The cranial base release technique was helpful in returning Amy's atlas to its original location. Regional tissue release was also performed on the neck, followed by another cranial base release.

The day after Christmas Amy arrived and immediately reported that she was headache-free and had been able to enjoy a nice Christmas. I resurveyed her and found the parietal still bowed, but the amount of the bow had been greatly reduced. Her atlas was in its correct location. I began with a thoracic diaphragm followed by repeating the rest of the 10-Step Protocol. Upon a final survey I found that the parietals were no longer bowed, and the atlas was still back where it belonged.

Mary Jo later told me that Amy had suffered no more headaches to date and had canceled her appointment with the neurologist.

Brendanne Phillips, BS, CST
Titusville, Florida
CranioSacral Therapy Practitioner since 1998

Dental Work Becomes a Headache

Reuben is a fourteen-year-old boy who came to me for help with constant, debilitating headaches. A very bright A-minus student, he excelled in most areas, had a very supportive family and little social pressure.

Diagnosed with a slight overbite, Reuben had braces put on his teeth approximately one year prior to my seeing him. About two months later the headaches began. Within three months he had to be taken out of school and home-schooled because the headaches only increased in intensity and duration. The pediatrician attributed the headaches basically to stress.

At that point Reuben's parents sent him to two temporo-mandibular joint syndrome (TMJ) specialists who said he should be splinted and medicated for pain. One made him a night splint because he thought Reuben was clenching his teeth. None of these things gave the boy any relief.

The doctor then wanted to send him to physical therapy, but there was no basis for doing that. Reuben was next tested by a neurologist who also diagnosed stress. He prescribed muscle relaxants and heavy pain medication. None of the doctors ever asked what other medications had been prescribed.

Another doctor said it was not TMJ, but he did not look beyond that for the cause of the headaches. Reuben was sent to a massage therapist for relaxation treatment. On a scale of zero to ten, with zero being pain-free and ten emergency-room pain, he rated Reuben's headaches as a seven.

Reuben's mother began searching for answers on her own. She found a book about alternative methods to treat headaches. It mentioned CranioSacral Therapy and listed references in the back.

In our first conversation I asked her a number of questions. From her answers I was able to describe the type of pain Reuben was having. She set up an appointment to bring him in for an intensive at the clinic. This consisted of two hours a day of treatment for four days (a two-hour evaluation and six hours of treatment).

Upon initial evaluation I saw a typical fourteen-year-old boy of slender build, with marked forward head, upper cervical extension, and fascial restrictions throughout his body. His headaches would come and go and were mainly "cranial cap" headaches. He had no neck pain and minimal TMJ pain on the right, with popping at the joint only on opening the jaw.

I did a full assessment of Reuben's body to determine any additional imbalances. I found increased weight-bearing on the left lower extremity. His right iliac crest was higher. His left ASIS was forward and rotated down. The nipple line was asymmetrical, with the right side lower by approximately one inch. His right shoulder was lower than his left. The right clavicle at the sternoclavicular joint was more forward. His right ear was higher. The left PSIS was up. The left scapula was up and forward versus the right, which was lower and retracted. In a supine position both shoulders were significantly up off the mat, with the right more so than the left. He had no other pain besides the headaches.

Upon assessment of Reuben's intraoral cavity I found marked tightening of the pterygoids; the right was greater than the left. The vomer was very high up and immobile. It looked like his head had been placed in a vise. It was as though the sides had been compressed and everything was trying to come out the top of his head. His sphenoid was stuck and not moving. He had almost no cranial rhythm because of the immobility.

Reuben did very well with treatment. After the first session, the headache, which had been constant for the previous six months, was gone. The clicking and popping in the right side of his jaw had stopped, and he said he felt he could breathe better out of both sides of his nose.

I worked to balance the whole body and restore the craniosacral rhythm in order to ensure that the other CranioSacral Therapy adjustments would hold.

We achieved our goals. On his last visit, everything was balanced and aligned in a more neutral position. We had restored his craniosacral rhythm. We gave him some home exercises, along with posture and body mechanics training, so he could continue to progress. We instructed the parents that a growth spurt might cause some additional symptoms, but I could do more adjustments at that time.

Reuben was entirely pain-free after the second visit, and when he left he was standing in a more upright, balanced posture with significant improvement in his forward head posturing. He stopped using the night splint after our second visit because he was no longer clenching his teeth at night. When he left, he had a great big grin on his face because he was finally pain-free.

Since Reuben lives out of state, we called to follow up with him two weeks later. He reported that he was still pain-free and it was now easier for him to move in space. He will be returning to school to finish the semester with his friends, like a normal fourteen-year-old boy. We will see him periodically during school breaks for maintenance.

Frankie L. Burget, OTR, RMT
Bedford, Texas
CranioSacral Therapy Practitioner since 2003

Reading Skills Improve with CST

❀ A few years ago I was involved with a group of Healing Touch students who met twice a month in a local church to offer free community sessions. The idea was to use the experience to deepen our knowledge in our newly gained skills.

One Saturday morning a young girl and an elderly woman sat in one of the pews awaiting their turn. When I approached the lady to let her know that she was next, I was surprised to learn that it was the girl, her granddaughter, for whom they wanted help.

Eight-year-old Jeannie★ seemed unable to concentrate on her school work. Subsequently, her grades were below what Grandma felt she was capable of. Jeannie's mother had addiction issues and thus Jeannie was raised by Grandma, who also took care of other family members.

Jeannie was eager to please Grandma and readily climbed onto the massage table. She tried to lie still but was itchy and twitchy and had her eyes wide open observing her surroundings carefully. I immediately started doing CranioSacral Therapy (CST) rather than Healing Touch. Before I even got to work on Jeannie's head, she had her eyes closed and her body was calmer.

I proceeded with what I felt to be the appropriate protocol for this child. Within a few minutes she was totally relaxed and hardly spoke a word. I spoke mentally to her body, telling her that all was safe, she was much loved, and she could relax in her life and do what she came to do.

When Jeannie returned two weeks later, I repeated pretty much the same protocol, again being drawn to do CST on her. A month later, Grandma reported that Jeannie's reading was better and that her report card showed improvement. On the following visit, the last time I saw them, Jeannie was enjoying reading and was doing much more of it than before.

★ Name changed to protect patient confidentiality

Eliane A. Viner, RN
Durango, Colorado
CranioSacral Therapy Practitioner since 1998

James's Choice

When I first met James, he was nine months old. He had been born three months prematurely and weighed one and a half pounds. He spent the first ten weeks of his life in the neonatal intensive care unit (NICU) of the hospital, where he showed steady progress.

The James I met was a beautiful, healthy little boy whose growth and development were generally appropriate. The only major concern was that he was not using his arms or hands at all. His hands remained fisted and held rigidly against his chest, with virtually no active or passive range of motion present. On a previous assessment by another physical therapist, James was considered to have a tight shoulder girdle, and his mother was told that he would likely benefit from physical therapy.

As a licensed physical therapist, I was asked to see and treat James. His mother was not familiar with CranioSacral Therapy (CST), so I explained it to her. James and I spent a total of one hour together that day.

With Mom and another staff member present, I sat on the floor with James in my arms. As my hands felt and worked to release the fascial tension throughout his chest and shoulder girdle, I began an inaudible heart-to-heart, soul-to-soul "dialogue" with him. I silently congratulated him on being such a remarkable survivor. As this dialogue continued, I had a feeling that James' posturing of his hands and arms was protective in nature.

I tried to imagine what it would be like to be so tiny and defenseless in the hands of so many strangers while undergoing so many procedures. Was his contracted posture one of fear? We talked about how his circumstances had changed. He was no longer in the NICU but at home with his wonderfully loving parents and older siblings. I asked him if he felt safe now. I also asked him if he would like to be in control of his upper extremities and make choices about how he used his arms and hands—to play, to feed himself, or to provide protection, security, and self-comfort.

At this point in the CST session, James' six-year-old brother Peter came home from school. He was curious to know what this stranger was doing with his baby brother. As I held James in my arms, I had Peter kneel by my side so that he was looking down into James' face. Then, for the first time in his life, James reached out. He stretched his arms over his head and began to touch and explore his brother's face.

On my next visit the following week, Mom reported that James was reaching out to grab everything. He was also sleeping with his arms stretched up over his head. He continued to freely use his arms and hands after that one CST session. Mom said, "I will always remember that day. It was amazing, touching, unbelievable."

James is now three and a half years old. His mother says he is doing great, and his progress is age-appropriate in all areas of development.

Veronica Quarry, MSPT
Arlington, Massachusetts
CranioSacral Therapy Practitioner since 1996

The Body's Wisdom and CST

❁ There are so many stories to tell of how CranioSacral Therapy has changed the lives of people of all ages and conditions. Here are four of my favorite.

A twenty-month-old girl was brought to me for help with chronic ear infections that had begun at eight months of age. Doctors had put her on antibiotics, but the infections always returned after the treatment stopped.

In our first session I noticed that the girl had discomfort and tightness around T3-4 [thoracic vertebrae]. She would not stay still until I did the ear pull, then she lay still for about forty-five minutes. Her mother said that she had never seen her be so quiet. If I moved my hands from her ear she would start to jump all around the room. I therefore stayed with the ear pull until I felt her body softening and she became absolutely still.

On the girl's second visit, just over four months later, her mother said that she had not had an infection since the first session, was less irritable, and was a much happier child. This time around she only allowed me to work on her for about thirty minutes. I focused on her neck and throat, releasing any restrictions I found.

The girl's third visit, about two months later, lasted about fifteen minutes. The mother reported that her daughter had experienced no ear infections and was doing very well. Some three years later this had not changed. The girl has never had another ear infection since our first treatment.

A fifty-two-year-old woman came to see me with pain on the left side of her rib cage around ribs seven, eight, and nine. She had been having this pain for three months. The pain was only at night when she tried to sleep on that side, and was so bad it would wake her up.

Around that same time the woman had an abnormal mammogram of the left breast. In my evaluation I found an energy cyst on her rib cage and some restriction around the breast area. I did diaphragm releases and an energy cyst release, following the tissue until I felt there were no restrictions.

A second mammogram three days later showed only normal tissue. She has had no pain in her rib cage since then and sleeps through the night.

A thirty-one-year-old woman came to see me after a car accident. She was complaining about discomfort in her neck and back. During evaluation, using the cranial rhythm, fascial glide, and arcing, I found restrictions in her neck, head, and back, and an energy cyst in her left foot. I asked her about her foot, since she did not mention it as one of the places of pain from the car accident.

She said the pain in her foot had begun while on vacation. She was wearing flip-flops while walking when she started having pain in her arch. On the following day she had sharp pain in the big toe, which radiated into the arch and the ankle joint. Because of the pain she started to limp and had to stop running.

That first session consisted of work on her head, neck, spine, and sacrum, along with a regional tissue release (unwinding) of the big toe and ankle. The pain in her toe immediately decreased.

After the second visit the woman was able to complete a twenty-six-mile hike with some toe stiffness, but no pain. After the third visit she had good joint mobilization and no pain. It took a few more visits to work out the neck and back injury, but she is doing well and is very happy to be able to go back to her regular routines of work and exercise.

My grandniece April was born with a heart problem. She only has two heart chambers and no pulmonary vessels. I only see her once a year since she lives in New York and I live in California. When she was born the doctors said they could not give her medication or operate on her, and she would not live past the age of eight years.

April is now ten years old. When she was younger, she did not like me to work on her. As she got older, though, she enjoyed it and now asks for it. I work on her every year when I go home.

In 2002 my sister mentioned that April's lips kept turning purplish when she played. I did diaphragm releases focusing on the hyoid and thoracic inlet. The next day my sister said April was fine. She has seldom had the problem since then.

In 2003, while I was attending a class in New York, I had the opportunity to work on April with two other CranioSacral Therapists: Aria Rose and Elyze Stewart.

A few months later, at April's regular checkup, her doctors wanted to know if surgery had been done because there was a change in her heart flow. They put April on medication and said there was a possibility that surgery could be performed.

I saw April this year (2004), and she asked me to work on her nose and other parts of her body. She understands that the body can heal itself, and that, with the help of bodywork and medicine, she can have a happy, healthy life.

Dusa Althea Rammessirsingh, BA, CMT, CST
San Francisco, California
CranioSacral Therapy Practitioner since 1986

CST Helps Learning-Disabled Children

CranioSacral Therapy (CST) has reached a school system in Northern Alberta. On four occasions I went to Saddle Lake, a Cree nation with some five thousand–plus natives, located in a rural area about an hour and a half from Edmonton. Unemployment there is high, and many people are on welfare. Drugs and alcohol are a continual problem. Some very well-educated and dedicated people work in the elementary school with four hundred and fifty students. I had the occasion to provide CranioSacral Therapy to seven of those students.

The occasion presented itself following a lecture that another therapist and I made at a teachers convention. The vice-principal of the school, who was in attendance, invited me to speak to his staff along with the parents of children he thought might benefit from CranioSacral Therapy. These parents generously agreed to entrust their children to my touch.

Five-year-old Blair★ was my first client. Accompanied by his mother, he walked shyly into the room. At school he usually did not make it past nine-thirty in the morning before being sent to the office crying. He was violent with the other children, and his attention span was about one minute. He was prescribed Ritalin, which his mother was reluctant to give him. I managed to apply all of the 10-Step Protocol, except for the techniques that involved the sacrum. The session lasted fifty-five minutes, which was awesome in itself. After Blair's third session, the school reported that he had not been to the office, and he had received the "Most Improved Student" award.

Ivan★ was an eleven-year-old who was very wary of the "white woman." He had only one lung, and his heart was on the wrong side. He was in great pain, but this was normal to him since he had

---

★Names changed to protect client confidentiality

lived with it since birth. After our first session, he looked at me with tears of relief in his eyes and thanked me over and over again. After our third session he said he felt even better.

Six-year-old Kelsey★ had fallen down two sets of stairs when he was four and had since experienced numerous other falls. He could not sit still and had behavior difficulties. After just one CST session he said that he no longer had headaches, backaches, or trouble sleeping; he felt very good.

Edward,★ a seven-year-old, complained of headaches that made him throw up. He also said he felt frustrated in school. Soon after our CST session, he let me know that he had received a perfect score on his spelling test. Before CST, he never would have been able to concentrate long enough to even take the test.

How wonderful that this school saw the relevance of Cranio-Sacral Therapy in not only improving their students' school work, but in changing their whole lives. I look forward to receiving word on how they are all doing. I also eagerly await further invitation to treat these beautiful children. They are unique and precious pebbles that have started a ripple effect that I hope will continue on to other schools and children throughout our area and the world.

Judy Pszyk
Bonnyville, Alberta, Canada
CranioSacral Therapy Practitioner since 2000

Follow the Example

❀ I'm a pediatric physical therapist whose treatment approach has been drastically altered by the use of CranioSacral Therapy (CST). Over the years there have been so many success stories. It took me a long time to consider who among my clients was most impacted by CST.

I thought of the girl who, at fourteen months old, had never rolled over, crawled, or pulled to stand. She was able to sit and was starting to scoot on her bottom. She had been extracted at birth through an emergency vacuum procedure, thus putting her life force at the top of her head. Through CST and parent education she progressed nicely through all the developmental stages. The day she was discharged four months later, she ran across the room to me.

Or should I choose the eight-year-old boy with cerebral palsy who only had two phrases: "Yeah" and "Go to gra-ma's"? Now the most common phrase I hear is, "Ellen, please go home." He also says a lot of other things: He recites the alphabet; he requests a variety of foods he wants to eat; and he spells his name.

What about the twenty-one-year-old man with cerebral palsy who had such severe deformities the doctors were reluctant to recommend spinal surgery because it would most likely paralyze him? After only six weeks of CST, once per week, he was taller, and the pressure mark from his posterior rib cage resting on his pelvis was gone. Today he is able to take deep breaths and even lie on his stomach.

Or there's the four-year-old boy with the floppiest body I've ever seen. He now loves his adapted tricycle and is even taking steps in his walker.

How could I forget the tight, little baby who had a trach, was on oxygen, was G-tube fed, and had no real diagnosis? One of the most enjoyable aspects of his progress has been seeing the medical specialists rendered speechless as they watch this two-year-old boy cruising along furniture and starting to swallow.

Oh, and did I forget to mention that the moms of these last two boys have taken the first CranioSacral Therapy class, and one is signed up for the second level? How's that for impact?

Of all my cases, I think I've been most intrigued by the preemies, some born as young as twenty-three weeks. How can they survive or function when they come out so early? CranioSacral Therapy in these little ones is truly pure energy. I spend many treatments with goose bumps all over due to the energy exchange that occurs when holding these precious miracles in my hands.

Another very interesting aspect through all this has been the change in attitudes of my coworkers. Initially they didn't know about CST, and didn't want to. Now I have coworkers who are planning to take the course and are requesting that I treat their clients with CST.

So, whom do I choose? It would have to be me! I realize that as each family has been touched, so have I. Going into each case, I pray for the miracle of healing, realizing that only God could make a body with such a complex self-healing mechanism. Then I remember my religious teachings, that we're all supposed to follow the example of Jesus. Does that mean only to be nice to each other, or does it mean to strive to be a healer by tapping into God's pure energy? What an opportunity I've been handed! I understand that it's not my hands making the changes; they're only the instruments. It's that wonderful energy from above and around us that is being used to heal these precious beings.

Ellen Smith-Susan, PT
Mentor, Ohio
CranioSacral Therapy Practitioner since 1996

CranioSacral Therapy
and Adults

As your ability to trust increases, the voices that guide you can speak more softly.
—*John E. Upledger, DO, OMM*

CST Derails Accident's Effects

Judy Gray: Since having a profound personal experience in my first CranioSacral Therapy class more than ten years ago, this work has been my love and passion. I have had many gratifying experiences that I could write about; however, I have chosen the story of my client Caroline Haddock to share with you. It is a miracle. I prefer that you read this primarily in her own words.

Caroline: On June 15, 2002, while driving to my cabin on the farm where I'd had my office for fifteen years, I began to cross the unmarked railroad tracks, well-covered by summer's outburst of overhanging trees. Only in brief flashbacks do I recall the barreling nose of the freight train that bored into my car on the passenger side at forty-five miles per hour.

The force crushed my 1982 Mercedes Benz bite by bite under its iron wheels, coming within a fraction of my elbow as it pushed me a thousand feet down the track. The windshield imploded into my body. Though I was in an altered state and had sustained multiple fractures, I managed to release myself from the seat belt, frog-kick myself out through the open windshield, and land in the gravel just before the train devoured the remnants of my vehicle.

I was helicoptered to the hospital, and my story was featured on the eleven o'clock news and front page of the local newspaper. After seeing this, those who knew me gave me up for dead, or at least permanently and severely disabled.

At my insistence, Judy Gray, co-owner, instructor, and therapist at the Lexington Healing Arts Academy, agreed to take me on as a client within a week of my accident. I had watched the work this group did with my infant grandson two weeks after he suffered compression and trauma during delivery. He was completely healed.

Judy: At first when Caroline came to me I was very reluctant to work on her because it was so soon after such a massive trauma. She was very insistent, and I finally agreed to just put my hands on her for an evaluation. I told her that she must have some huge angels that really wanted her to stay here to do something. It felt like the treatment room filled up to capacity. I was very moved and surprised to feel the trauma in her nervous system while feeling the amazing calm in her at the same time. She always went into such a relaxed state that there was no resistance in her body to the treatment.

Caroline: As a clinical social worker in private practice for thirty years, I have much experience in dealing with inner healing of trauma memories, anxiety, depression, and related areas. In all those years I had never seen such a dramatic shift from release work.

My internist, a distinguished graduate of Johns Hopkins University, warned me against using such alternative methods. He continued to send me to orthopedic surgeons and neurosurgeons for my closed-head injury. He also continued to medicate the pain I was experiencing from the blow to my spinal column caused by more than four hundred tons of weight crashing into me at forty-five miles per hour. I had no use of either arm for two months. My cranium and jaw were compressed, and TMJ had developed. I was receiving round-the-clock care.

Judy's work often left me in a trancelike state, which always felt relieving. It somehow helped me bypass the expected development of serious depression and frequent flashbacks and trauma-related nightmares. She instructed me on how to use the Still Point Inducer at my home. The energy in my body began to work synergistically to not only heal current wounds but past wounds of trauma memories. It was a prayer answered, as knots began to unravel and energy was unbound so that physical wounds could resolve.

This has not only amazed me from the standpoint of my psychiatric training, but it has bewildered my medical doctors and associates. Instead of thinking that I am special, I am directing them to believe that this process of CranioSacral Therapy is valid and must be documented scientifically and covered by medical insurance. If others can have access to this healing, it can speed recovery immeasurably and reduce suffering for all who are blocked and need the doors reopened. Is this not the goal of the medical arts and healing?

Judy: I have seen Caroline every week for two years now. It took almost a full year for her energetic and physical bodies to come fully into alignment. At present I find that she needs the consistent tune-up to keep her aligned. She continues to have some difficulty with short-term memory, and yet she is fully functional in her work and her life. Caroline has been such a joy and inspiration for me to have as a client. Her spirit is full of light and acceptance.

Caroline: Today, two years later, I am the essence of a medical and spiritual miracle. I primarily thank God, my loved ones, an intense will to live, and CranioSacral Therapy for my strong recovery.

Story by Caroline Haddock
Submitted by Judy Gray, LMT
Lexington, Kentucky
CranioSacral Therapy Practitioner since 1992

Seeing Isn't Believing, Believing Is Seeing

Ralph was a fifty-two-year-old junior high school history teacher. He came to see me at the urging of his wife Beverly, who was a client. Ralph was very skeptical that CranioSacral Therapy (CST) could help him with his problem.

"I do not have any problem believing Beverly feels better," he said. "She sings praises about how this therapy fixes her back. But it's my eye. What can you do with my eye?" Then he looked at me seriously and added: "You're not going to massage my eyeball, are you?!"

Ralph explained that the week prior, his ophthalmologist had told him that his only functioning eye (the left eye was blinded as a child in a BB gun accident) was showing signs of macular degeneration. He understood the doctor to say that the progression of the degeneration seemed to be especially aggressive.

Ralph loved teaching, and the students at this rural junior high school loved Ralph. He was hoping to put off retirement at least until his youngest daughter got through college, but now it looked like he would be retiring at the end of the current semester. He also had a passion for reading, and that was already being severely compromised.

Ralph's skepticism, as well as his ever-increasing depression and anger about his eyesight, was getting the best of him. He wanted to have hope, but he felt hopeless. He agreed to let me do CST with him for only thirty minutes after his wife's appointment. According to Beverly, this was quite a concession for him.

After briefly explaining the anatomy of the cranial system, I did some arcing. Ralph's body wanted to focus on the sphenobasilar joint. I began with a thoracic diaphragm release and occipital-cranial base release. I followed that with a frontal and parietal lift.

Next I focused on the sphenobasilar joint. I spent fifteen minutes evaluating and treating any cranial base dysfunctions that his body showed me. The most profound dysfunction of the sphenobasilar joint appeared to be compression. The session was completed with an L5/S1 decompression and a dural tube rock and glide.

Ralph had fallen asleep. When he awoke, he reported feeling more energized. His wife thought his eyes and skin color looked brighter, too. After a few minutes, however, Ralph reported that his sight remained unchanged. I told him that changes could continue to happen over the next week and to keep in touch. He decided not to reschedule for further treatment.

Six days later, I got a phone call from Beverly telling me to expect a call from him. She had an appointment scheduled the next day and wanted me to know that Ralph might be coming with her. I did not hear from him, but he was the first one in the door the next day. He could not wait to tell me what had happened.

Ralph said he had been driving his pickup truck through town when all of a sudden he heard a "pop" in his head. He started realizing that the vision in his right eye had changed. Colors were brighter and images were becoming sharper. He was close to his ophthalmologist's office, so he pulled in. As is typical of a small rural town doctor's office, Ralph walked in, waved to the receptionist (who was probably a former student), and caught the doctor in the hallway.

After hearing how Ralph's sight had changed, the doctor decided to rerun the tests he had done two weeks prior. The second tests showed no signs of macular degeneration, and the doctor told him the first test results must have been wrong. Ralph did not feel confident enough to tell the doctor he had received CranioSacral Therapy six days before; he just said that he knew there had been a change in his vision.

Ralph came back to see me because, as he put it, "If it was this stuff that did it, I want to make sure it sticks."

Ralph received six more half-hour sessions in which we addressed more restrictions in the dural membrane and worked to normalize a triad compression. After the third session, Ralph reported that the pain he had had in his left eye since the BB gun accident was gone. (The BB is still lodged by Ralph's left optic nerve.)

Ralph's daughter finished college, and two years later Ralph retired. He and Beverly now enjoy traveling between the homes of their three daughters and have become new grandparents. Ralph says he has the most beautiful granddaughter ever.

Ultimately, Ralph did not know what to believe, which goes to prove that it is not essential to "believe" anything specific with this work. Ralph had the heart and the strong desire to live life to the fullest. His body's wisdom knew how to make that happen.

Do I need to know how it happened? Did the releases provide for more blood circulation? Did they work out restrictions in the membranes or optic nerve? How about the increasing cerebrospinal fluid movement? What was the "pop" all about? Could it be all of the above, none of the above, or something else altogether? I may never be absolutely sure. Ralph's doctor did not know. And, to be honest, Ralph doesn't care. It worked!

Lauri J. Rowe, MA, NCTMB, CST-D
Coldwater, Michigan
CranioSacral Therapy Practitioner since 1998

Pastor Dan, Man of Faith

※ Our new pastor got sick shortly after coming to our church. He was having migraines and upper respiratory problems. I barely knew him, but I finally got the courage to suggest that CranioSacral Therapy (CST) might help. I was uncertain how he would receive my suggestion. When I broached the topic, he showed some interest and accepted my offer to work on him.

I wanted him to have confidence in me and in CST, so as part of my explanation of the work I told him that it is scriptural, like laying on of hands. I was caught off guard by his response. He looked at me from across his desk and said, "Well, that sounds nice, but is there any empirical data to support its effectiveness?" I had expected a less technical question from a man of faith. Apparently, though, I was able to explain the physiological aspects of CST to his satisfaction, because he agreed to let me work on him.

In the first session I arced to his respiratory diaphragm, which was higher than I had expected in a tall man with a long torso. The first release was rather dramatic. After just a few seconds, he took a deep gasp of air, and I felt his breathing drop from his chest to his abdomen. I also felt a shift in his diaphragm. As it released, it seemed to relax and drop lower in his chest, freeing up his breathing. He commented that he could feel air deeper in his lungs than he had for some time. There was a corresponding softening and opening in the thoracic outlet. His hyoid responded nicely, allowing for opening in the throat and deepening of his voice.

Pastor Dan's presenting complaint had been persistent migraine headaches. When I monitored the cranial rhythm, I felt a restriction of the flow to the left. Similarly, I found restrictions on the left side of the frontal bone, the sphenoid, the parietals, and the temporal bones. I didn't know which side was affected by his headaches, so I asked if they were primarily on the left. He was surprised that I was able to identify the affected side. When I did a

CV-4 still point, he went very quickly into a deep still point. I was somewhat alarmed by its depth and duration. When the rhythm came back on, he was not only more relaxed, but he noted a total relief from the constant pressure on the left side of his head. He said he hadn't realized how much tension he had been holding until it was gone.

Knowing that he had had a recent root canal, I suggested that he might benefit from some mouth work in his next session. I explained the avenue of expression. Since speaking is an important aspect of his work, and he had already experienced an opening up in his throat, he agreed to give it a try.

Pastor Dan's next session came sooner than expected. When he was too sick to come to church on Sunday, I called to tell him that I was coming over. He was mildly resistant to the idea but agreed that if it would help him feel better, he'd give it a try.

When I arrived I found that he had been very sick, running a high fever, coughing until his chest ached, and unable to get out of bed. He had been to the doctor, who diagnosed flu with a possible secondary infection in the bronchi. The doctor prescribed antibiotics, which resulted in vomiting and abdominal cramping.

My approach was very basic. A series of still points helped lower the fever. Work to the respiratory diaphragm allowed for deeper and less strained breathing. Gentle traction of the dural tube revealed a restriction in the thoracic area that seemed to correspond to the aching in his chest. And dural tube rock and glide led to a softening and lengthening of the paravertebral and intercostal muscles, resulting in less chest pain.

I finished the session with another still point, then advised his wife that I expected he would sleep more comfortably. She later told me that he had slept soundly for five hours, after which he reported that he was feeling better and was hungry. His illness ran its course in another couple of weeks, leaving him pale, weak, and listless but able to resume his regular schedule.

After he seemed well enough, I once more presented the idea of a session with mouth work. Again he seemed somewhat skeptical but willing to give it a try.

The session went very well. He experienced a widening in the maxillae, a relief of restriction in the left palatine, and improved synchrony of the sphenoid and vomer rhythm. Releasing the zygoma relieved sinus pressure. At the end of the session he told me that he felt like he was breathing in areas previously unavailable to him.

After only three sessions, he reports that he is feeling great, has no more headaches, is breathing much easier, and has a lot more support for his voice when he preaches.

I don't know if this experience has strengthened Pastor Dan's faith, but I guess he has become a believer in CranioSacral Therapy.

Lynne Tupper, MPH, OTR, CST
Houston, Texas
CranioSacral Therapy Practitioner since 1998

Athlete Finds New Life After Career-Ending Stroke

❀ On July 30, 1991, twenty-eight-year-old Jeff Gray, a relief pitcher for the Boston Red Sox, suffered a career-ending stroke. It affected the right side of his body and was caused by a congenital blood vessel abnormality in his head—a mere three-millimeter piece of tissue that restricted the flow of blood to his brain.

For the first two hours after the stroke, Jeff had total right-sided paralysis. Doctors worried that he would never walk again, let alone throw a baseball. He spent the next ten days in a Boston-area hospital and one night in a rehabilitation center before beginning outpatient care. After his discharge he returned to his home in Bradenton, Florida.

I had just moved to Bradenton from Canada when Jeff started therapy at the clinic where I was working. He received conventional treatment consisting of range-of-motion and other therapeutic exercises. The clinic staff had never heard of CranioSacral Therapy and were very skeptical of it. I believed, however, that CST would help release some of the scar tissue in Jeff's brain, improve circulation, reduce muscle tone, and allow the brain to heal, which would result in a return of functional movements. When I explained this to Jeff, he was very motivated to try it.

When he showed up for our first appointment, his wife Claire had to help him in and out of the car. Wearing a brace on his right foot and ankle, Jeff struggled to walk with a cane. Initial evaluation indicated increased muscle tone in the right side of Jeff's body, limited range of motion, very little use of his right foot and hand, little movement in his arm and leg, and increased neurological tone in his shoulder and leg. His speech was slurred, and he had very little strength.

Our first goal was to make Jeff a functional human being again—able to walk without a cane, sign his own name, dress and bathe himself, drive himself to the clinic, and exercise independently.

I developed a program whereby Jeff would receive CranioSacral Therapy daily to reduce the muscle tone on the right side of his body, reduce any scar tissue in the brain and spinal cord, and improve circulation. My thinking was that if CranioSacral Therapy were to have an effect, we would see a change in his functional activities, range of motion, and strength. At that point, we would work on his fine-motor skills, followed by aerobic work and strength training.

Within three months, Jeff was performing as a functional human being. He could do all the things listed above, except pitch in the major leagues. I remember meeting the team doctor at the Tampa Airport. While he was very pleased about Jeff's improvements, he cautioned him not to expect more; that was probably as far as he could get. This was the response of most people. I, on the other hand, was ecstatic for him. We had achieved our first goal: to be a functional human being again.

Most people would be happy reaching that goal, but not Jeff. After seeing the gains he had made to that point, he kept pushing. He still wanted to play baseball again. We made a new goal to prepare him to return to baseball by the middle of the next season. Our workouts intensified.

In order to pitch again, Jeff would need full use of his fingers as well as his foot for pushing off the pitcher's mound. Our intention was to free up the scar tissue, improve circulation, and help his brain regenerate as much as possible. Then we would introduce functional movements and teach his brain how to throw a ball and move again like a baseball player. He would continue with fine-motor exercises for his hands.

As Jeff gained strength each week, we elevated his workouts. It got to where he was training six hours a day. He would begin each morning at home working on manual dexterity: typing four or five paragraphs from the newspaper, writing letters, and stuffing envelopes. Upon arrival at the clinic, he would receive CranioSacral Therapy for one to two hours. Then he would spend an hour weight–lifting followed by the bike, Stairmaster, Versa climber, and treadmill.

Soon Jeff had progressed from throwing a Nerf ball to throwing a baseball about fifteen to twenty feet.

CranioSacral Therapy worked extremely well for Jeff. He progressed very quickly with his gross- and fine-motor skills. Each week he got stronger, faster, more mobile, more flexible, and more coordinated. The degree of his improvement was far above the initial predictions and expectations of Jeff's doctors, other therapists, coaches, and friends.

By February 1992 we had advanced Jeff to a pitcher's mound, where he was throwing the full distance at approximately seventy miles per hour. Tests conducted in Boston that same month showed that his brain had regenerated to replace the damaged area, and new blood vessels had grown and were serving the brain matter. In addition, the abnormality had shrunk, which baffled doctors. They had predicted that it would stay the same, at best. They did not understand how that had happened.

By our last session together, Jeff was speaking normally. He could walk, run, sign his name, play golf, and throw a baseball. He was stronger, had less body fat, and was more mobile, flexible, and faster than he had been before the stroke. He was throwing the ball at ninety miles per hour and jogging two to three miles a day. He eventually went back to professional baseball for a ten–year stint as a pitching coach. He is now a financial advisor and has a son who is playing baseball. Jeff credits CranioSacral Therapy with allowing him to enjoy a fulfilling life and continue to play catch with his son.

Kerry D'Ambrogio, PT, DOM
Bradenton, Florida
CranioSacral Therapy Practitioner since 1993

In the Pits

✽ It was Christmastime, and I had just finished taking the second-level CranioSacral Therapy class, where I learned the mouth protocol. Little did I know how quickly that knowledge would come in handy.

I was at a Christmas party when the pit of a date got lodged in the roof of my mouth. It was positioned horizontally, from the left inner side to the right inner side of my upper teeth. I could not talk because the pit was in the way of my tongue.

I motioned to my friend who was with me and showed him what had happened. He attempted to pull the pit out, but all it did was hurt. It felt like he was pulling my teeth out along with part of my face.

I then had a visual flashback to the class where I learned the movement of the maxilla. I decided to try applying this new information to my predicament.

I found a place where no one was around, for I was a bit concerned how it would look having both my hands inside my mouth. I first calmed myself down by inducing a still point. I then began to tune into the flexion/extension movement of the maxilla.

As I tuned in, facilitating the widening of the maxilla and relaxing more, I noticed that the grip my upper teeth had on the pit began to loosen. This continued until the widening was enough for the pit to come completely out of its lodged position. Balancing my sphenoid and inducing another still point allowed me to rejoin and enjoy the party.

Maria Scotchell, BA, RMT
Austin, Texas
CranioSacral Therapy Practitioner since 1997

Another Skeptic Converts to CST

❀ My husband, a retired Marine and a "show me the money" kind of guy, was one of my first clients after I completed my initial CranioSacral Therapy class. He was completely skeptical.

While I was working on his sacral area, following the 10-Step Protocol with careful precision, he experienced pain in his left knee. (This is a man who has a high degree of pain tolerance.) At the same time, I was feeling powerful pulsing in his lower back. Leaving the sacrum area, I went to the head and neck. I was drawn, however, to return to the lower back area. Again he experienced severe pain and discomfort in his knee. At that point I ended the session, feeling that he needed time to process the whole experience.

An hour later, we were together in the computer room, and I went to the kitchen to get some water. When I returned, my husband had the oddest look on his face. I asked what was happening.

He replied, "I was just sitting here and I felt this strange sensation in my lower back that moved up my spine. I was wondering if I should even move. Then it traveled up my back, following my spine. When it reached my upper back it felt just like a 'bubble.' It kept moving, up to my shoulder and my neck, and then in a 'poof' it went out my left ear."

I asked him what he did next.

"I was afraid to move, but I did slowly." Then he looked at me and said smiling, "The pain was completely gone. I'm pain-free— my whole back, leg, and knee!"

Because he never complains, I asked him how long he had been in this pain. There was a long pause, and he said two years.

Since that time I've completed my second CranioSacral Therapy class and have been using this modality ever since.

Susan Tveit, CMT
Lemoore, California
CranioSacral Therapy Practitioner since 2003

Climbing the Mountain

❀ In September of 2000, Brent was thrown from his bike into a ditch while on a scenic touring ride in the White Mountains. Though he wore a helmet, the impact was severe enough to result in a closed-head mild traumatic brain injury. The official medical diagnosis was a left frontal intraventricular hematoma. In addition, he sustained a fractured left clavicle and right radius.

Brent was initially treated at a local hospital but was soon airlifted to Maine Medical Center. En route the EMT initiated a ventriculostomy, and Brent was intubated to maximize oxygen intake. He spent five days in the ICU followed by one week at a rehabilitation hospital.

While at the rehab center, Brent began a plan of treatment that included speech, occupational, and neuropsychological therapies. He was on a leave of absence from his job for about three months following the accident, and spent the next six months on a managed back-to-work plan administered by a neuropsychologist.

Brent continued to experience almost total amnesia of the two weeks following the accident. Although issues with short-term memory improved slowly over the two years following the accident, he continued to experience residual effects.

I first saw Brent in the beginning of February 2001, five months after his accident. Our intake interview was an overview of the accident (or as much of it as he could remember) and a review of any treatments that he had or was presently receiving. His major complaint at the time was a feeling of dizziness and memory problems.

As soon as I placed my hands on Brent's feet to arc his body, it was obvious that the left and right sides of his body were one hundred eighty degrees out of phase with each other. Arcing, as one might surmise, pointed directly to the temporal bones. One side was going into flexion while the other side was moving into extension.

At this point, I went through a 10-Step Protocol to balance his body and assess if the problem areas could be isolated. Since no firsthand facts were available to me, it was beneficial to gather as much information as possible.

Once we completed the temporal bone techniques, symmetry returned to a normal pattern, rhythm was a little on the low end of normal range, and amplitude was weak. These symptoms didn't surprise me since it was easy to assume that he had been in this asymmetrical pattern since the accident; however, I really had no way of knowing.

The next two sessions strengthened the foundation for Brent's continuing recovery. His symmetry was consistent, and the amplitude increased with each treatment.

Concurrent to these sessions, Brent was undergoing a series of ten Structural Integration treatments, along with cognitive, speech, and occupational therapies. Given his improved condition, we decided to hold off on more CST until he had completed his other therapies. If the dizziness or balance issues returned, he would come back sooner rather than later for more work.

The following are Brent's words regarding his CST experience:

"I remember the first session as being very relaxing (trancelike) but uneventful. After completing her assessment, Barbara asked if I had been experiencing any difficulty in executing motion that involved crossing my body. I had to admit that I had been dropping things with great frequency and having difficulty in coordinating motions that involved my left and right hands acting in concert. In addition, I felt that my walking had an 'out of control' aspect to it, but I had chalked it up to an equilibrium issue.

"I returned for two additional visits. After the second one, I was aware of greater confidence in my coordination while walking, a feeling of being better 'grounded.' During this second visit, I also started to execute what I can only assume was a remembered defensive motion with my left arm. Because I continue to have no recollection of the accident, it's impossible to say for sure, but since this is the side on which the clavicle fracture occurred, it seems a plausible explanation.

"Since early on in my recovery, I have been identified as a true success story. While it is impossible to attribute this to any single course of therapy, I am convinced that the reason why I have been able to return to my job, when so many with similar injuries are not, is that I was willing to avail myself of *all* forms of therapy. CranioSacral Therapy and massage used as adjuncts to the traditional therapies are why I am where I am today.

"While I may never understand how CST works, I no longer am skeptical of the benefits and have recommended it to others who are recovering from traumatic injuries."

As a therapist, I was amazed at the immediate and permanent results that CST produced over the first three treatments. Brent continues to experience regional tissue releases, which are giving his body more and more freedom as time goes on.

I am always humbled by this work and am in awe of the human potential to heal, whether it is through a conscious or nonconscious state, or, as I have come to learn, a combination of both.

I continue to see Brent for treatments. We are currently working out a maintenance plan.

Barbara May, CMT
Arlington, Massachusetts
CranioSacral Therapy Practitioner since 1994

CST Helps Body Self-Correct Trigeminal Neuralgia

It was a beautiful sunny morning that February as I walked on the beach. This was where I connected with God and found my strength and grounding abilities. That day I would have to draw from that strength, for Bob was coming to see me for the first time.

Sixty-nine-year-old Bob had been in pain for several years, suffering with trigeminal neuralgia. He had been to a number of doctors for this ailment. In the beginning, no one knew what he had. They sent him to a dentist, an oral surgeon, and a nutritionist, who finally told him about his trigeminal nerve.

Bob's pain grew to unbearable proportions. He went to Columbia Presbyterian Hospital in New York, where they did a procedure called Gamma Knife. During this procedure he had to remain motionless and wear a helmet of some sort while being given radiation to kill the nerve. Sadly, the treatment failed.

Bob was in so much excruciating pain that he couldn't touch his face and had to sleep in an upright position. He wasn't able to chew his food, so his wife pureed it and he sipped it through a straw. Not only was his quality of life greatly affected, he also had to take twelve hundred milligrams daily of Tegretol, a pain medication with nasty side effects that made his face blotchy and scaly.

One day Bob's wife Clara was having a reflexology session with a therapist who had just attended an Upledger Institute Cranio-Sacral Therapy (CST) workshop at which I was assisting. After Clara related her husband's pain to this woman, she suggested that they contact me.

To be honest, when I received the call I was apprehensive at best, wondering if I could help him. Yet with the trust and experience I have in CST, I thought it was worth the time and effort.

Bob arrived at my office with the help of Clara. He looked like a disturbed homeless man. He was wearing his pajama top because he couldn't pull a shirt over his head. His hair was matted because he could only wash it once a week. His face was blotchy and crusty. And his mouth had just a small opening. He shuffled into my office, mumbling to me how much pain he was feeling.

I brought him into my quiet massage room and sat him down. I placed one hand on his chest and the other on his back at the respiratory diaphragm, and just relaxed. Closing my eyes, I called in the energy and strength from the sun I had experienced that morning. My hands could feel the painful energy begin to release. I then moved up to the throat at the hyoid diaphragm, and I could feel his body relaxing. It almost felt like I was putting out the fire.

About twenty minutes into the session, I asked Bob if he wanted to lie down on the massage table. To his amazement, he thought he could. It had been six months since he had been able to lie down. While he was lying there, I began the direction-of-energy technique. My hands were drawn toward his chin, and from there toward his right cheek, then to the top of his lip. This is the area where the trigeminal nerve resides and where he felt the most pain. It was interesting how I could pick up the energy of the inflamed nerve.

Bob looked up at me and said, "Are you taking my pain?" I said, "No, it's coming out of your body, but it doesn't affect me." He said, "Good, I wouldn't want you to feel what I feel. How are you doing that?" I told him, "Your body is doing the work. I'm just assisting it."

He then started to move his mouth a little and realized there wasn't any pain. Then he opened his mouth for the first time in almost three months. He couldn't believe it. He realized that he was out of pain. He kept saying, "Oh, your hands are like angels' hands. How are you able to touch my face like this? It doesn't hurt me anymore!"

The truth was I had simply trusted in the work that Dr. Upledger taught me. I believe that the body has an innate way of healing itself. Sometimes all it needs is the right environment to activate the healing process. This was the right environment. And with faith on our side I was able to get Bob out of pain.

His session lasted about an hour. He sat up slowly and, while sitting on the edge of the table, he looked at me and said, "How did you do that? I can't believe I have been suffering so long. Why doesn't everybody know about this?"

I assured Bob that it wasn't me working alone. CranioSacral Therapy is a very powerful therapy, and it takes the patient and the therapist to spread the word about how it can help assist the body to correct itself.

Bob continued to come in weekly for seven weeks. I worked his cranial bones to correct some restrictions he had, which also helped his sinus problems. His wife lowered his Tegretol usage by one hundred milligrams a week.

At this writing, it is May. Bob now comes in every other week. He is free of pain and no longer takes the pain medication.

Nejie Miranda-Sylvester, CMT
Brick, New Jersey
CranioSacral Therapy Practitioner since 1993

Back Relief Without Rods, Screws, Nuts, or Bolts

✿ I enjoyed a wonderful Mother's Day today. I rode my horse in a Hunter Pace competitive race for ten miles. I would not have been able to do that two years ago.

At age sixty-five I am a very active person. I mow forty acres of our property, travel (often on genealogy projects), do bead work, and ride my Arabian horses.

In 2002 I was bucked off my horse. At the time I did not realize how bad the damage was. After a few months of pain and not being able to do the things I normally did, I went to a highly recommended sports orthopedic doctor.

The words I heard were not good. The only option I had to relieve the pain was surgery. When asked what the surgery consisted of, I was told that they would fuse three discs. There would be rods, screws, nuts, and bolts put into my back. To make things worse for a physically active person, the recovery period was at least six months, depending on how well I healed. Then there was the added "insult to injury" comment: The rods might have to be taken out at some later date.

When I asked what the chances were for me to be better, I didn't like that answer either. He said I would have one chance in four of being better. In other words, the likelihood was greater that I could be worse or see no difference at all. Those odds were not good enough for me to consider the surgery.

Unable to walk, stand for any length of time, or lift anything of any size, I had to hire someone to help me around the farm.

That's when a massage therapist I had been going to recommended that I see Christine Bennett. I started going to her about twice a week.

I began to feel relief from the pain almost immediately. Gradually I was able to shop without having to sit after only a few minutes, and to ride in a car without being in excruciating pain.

I also experienced an unexpected benefit related to a 1986 surgery I had undergone to repair a ruptured disc in my neck. At the time, the doctor had told me there was a possibility of some side effects. The one I remember the most was that my voice box could be damaged. When I asked what the percentage was of success, I was told ninety-nine percent—so I said go for it.

I didn't realize until six months after the surgery that my voice box had indeed been damaged. All I knew was that I was constantly clearing my throat as if I had sinus drainage. I kept a cough drop in my mouth just about all the time, as that seemed to help some. Since Christine began working on me, the throat problem has almost completely gone away.

After about a year and a half of seeing Christine, I am back to riding my horses and cutting my own grass. I can now travel by car and by plane with minimal discomfort.

I have become a one hundred percent believer in CranioSacral Therapy. I have taken an introductory CranioSacral Therapy class and plan to take the first full level of coursework sometime this year. I want to learn more about how to help myself and my family and friends.

I can still put myself in a situation where I have some pain, but now I know what to do to relieve it. If not for CranioSacral Therapy, I would definitely not be in the physical shape I am today.

Thank you, Christine, and thank you Upledger Institute for teaching Christine how to show me how to live.

Story by Peggy McMakin, client
Submitted by Christine Rydholm-Bennett, LMT, NCTMB
Wilmington, North Carolina
CranioSacral Therapy Practitioner since 1997

My Thoracic Inlet Experience

❀ Being a massage therapist, I know that I need to get bodywork on a regular basis to keep myself in the best shape possible. As such, I often try the services of therapists with whom I
have not previously worked.

One Friday evening I received a massage on my sore and aching
shoulders and upper back. I had never received a massage from this
therapist before. I specified that I was holding my tension in my
neck, shoulders, and upper back, and that this was the area I wanted
worked on. She proceeded to give me an okay massage. I felt
"worked over" afterwards, but I did feel a little looser.

The following day was Saturday, and I found myself with a headache coming on. Saturday is my day to relax, which is hard to do
with a headache. Not one to take painkillers, I am more inclined
to move around and see if a little activity, such as walking and gentle stretching, can relieve the situation. A night's sleep proved to be
the only thing that brought any relief. But relief was only temporary. By Sunday afternoon, my headache was still with me.

I don't know why, but something prompted me to ask my husband, a massage therapist trained in CranioSacral Therapy, to do a
thoracic inlet diaphragm release on me. I lay on the edge of the
bed and he put his hands on me to do the diaphragm release. He
worked on me for about two to three minutes, and I began to feel
things inside letting go and moving. After another minute or two I
told him he could finish.

When I got up, I experienced the most amazing sensation. It
felt as if a drain in my head had been clogged and had just been
opened up. I felt fluid and energy draining down out of my head.
It was as if a life-giving shower had been poured over my whole
being.

My entire body became more alive as all my fluids and energy
flowed more smoothly within me. I felt more connected and more

comfortable in general. I still had a slight residual headache, but that drained within a few hours.

That Sunday afternoon I asked myself why I hadn't done the thoracic inlet technique earlier. I knew full well that when a cranial base release is done, a thoracic inlet release should be done as well. But then I recalled that the massage therapist I visited hadn't done a cranial base release, so I shouldn't have had this problem.

Now I know that when a person has a strong massage like that on a tense neck, shoulders, and back, a thoracic inlet release is needed—just one more lesson learned in how profound and powerful CranioSacral Therapy can be. And the beauty is, it is so simple that anyone can provide this type of relief for their family and friends.

Sometimes clients are our teachers, and sometimes we learn things ourselves the painful way. The next massage I got ended with a thoracic inlet release, and I had no headache the next day.

Julie McKay, CMT, RBFP
Madison, Wisconsin
CranioSacral Therapy Practitioner since 1998

"Piecing" a Loved One Back Together

❀ On March 22, 2002, my life partner Carol fainted while visiting her mom in the hospital. Landing face down, her head
bounced twice on the cement floor. Seven of her upper teeth disappeared into the bone; the left condyle of her mandible broke;
and her left ear canal was severed.

She was taken immediately to the emergency room, but was
soon transferred to another medical center that served as the region's
trauma facility. Even though she had gone unconscious with the
fall, at no time in either hospital did any medical personnel address
the possibility of injury to her brain or cranium. Attention focused
on stitches (where her teeth had gone through her lower lip), surgery to bring her teeth down (which resulted in the loss of two
front teeth), and her ear. Carol had her jaw wired shut for about
sixty days.

Due to her acute situation, she was forced to stay in Seattle,
where the accident had occurred. Unfortunately, we lived in Hawaii.
As a result, I did not see her until she was strong enough to return
home on May 11.

Carol is an author and public speaker who thoroughly enjoys
being with people. On July Fourth of that year, we went to a celebration at a local hotel to give her a "people" fix. After about one
hour she had to return home. She then proceeded to sleep for the
next forty hours, getting up only long enough to drink and use the
bathroom. After that her health did not return to the state it was
in before the celebration.

Initially, my CranioSacral Therapy treatments consisted of a modified 10-Step Protocol. Many of the sessions were short ones that
began with opening of the throat area and then moved to the head.
Most of the time I held a position lightly and did not even invite the
bones to move. I sensed that this would have been too invasive to
her traumatized state. Thus, I moved very slowly during the treat-

ments. When I was at her head once, I began incorporating a full 10-Step Protocol. I only mentally invited her bones to move, however; I did not push, pull, or move them at all.

After many months of treatment—when Carol was finally able to put her head down for short periods—one of her favorite treatments was an energetic-type shiatsu, ending with CranioSacral Therapy on her head. This combination of treatments balanced and restored her head and body so profoundly that she was able to perform many more normal tasks during the day.

Here are Carol's own words about her experience:

"I believe the reason I am nearly one hundred percent healed from this traumatic head injury is the daily (sometimes twice-daily) CranioSacral Therapy I have received from Roy. Without his loving attention and healing skills, I would likely still be sleeping my life away.

"Before receiving a treatment my brain often feels weak and scattered, unable to hold a thought. Though I'm not sleepy, I know I must rest because all my bodily systems are shutting down.

"Once I recline, I sleep for hours; during the first year of recovery it was sometimes days. How do I describe my sensations? I feel perhaps as an infant would, only able to slowly roll over in my crib. I see the world out there but I can't reach it. I must be still.

"As Roy touches me, I feel the familiar, gentle sense of the fragments of my inner head and brain reconnecting, finding their way home. As Roy's hands touch my head or sacrum during a CranioSacral treatment I feel comforted and safe. It feels like I'm being carefully glued together piece by piece. Beneath the bones in my head I sense an easing back into wholeness. Whatever is disconnected slowly, quietly, and effortlessly begins to come together.

"Because of the dramatic difference in myself before and after CranioSacral Therapy, I believe I am years ahead of where I would be had I not had daily sessions.

"For a while I (we) attended a head injury support group. As fellow brain-injured people shared, I ached with the thought: If only you were getting CranioSacral Therapy, I bet you would be functioning so much more fully."

Roy Kincaid, LMT
Kailua Kona, Hawaii
CranioSacral Therapy Practitioner since 2001

Cowboy Up

✿ The chute gate opens and the bronc rears up, slamming the straddling cowboy against the metal pipe behind him. He then lunges out into the arena, bucks three times hard, and sends the flopping cowboy flying. Ryan, the nineteen-year-old cowboy with curly black hair, lies limp in the arena. He is hurt badly. I sense that his back is broken.

Endless minutes hang before Ryan is loaded into an ambulance and whisked away to the hospital in Bonnyville. He is transferred to Edmonton, one hundred fifty miles away, where they determine that he has no feeling from his knees down. I hear that he has a rod and two pins put in his spine.

Four weeks later, after receiving the okay from his doctor, I go to treat Ryan at the family ranch. He is out of the rehab hospital for the weekend. The prospect of being able to help him is so exciting, yet I am scared of what I might feel. I touch him and immediately choke up. The trauma is so overwhelming.

I force myself to settle and hesitantly feel. There it is, ever so minute, but there all the same—a craniosacral rhythm, first in the left leg then in the right. A few tears squeeze out of my eyes. Yay, he has a rhythm! His spinal column is not severed! Again excitement. Again I have to settle myself.

What should I do? It is way too soon to do the full 10-Step Protocol of CranioSacral Therapy. I determine that diaphragm releases are the priority. The most obvious problems I start with are the torn mesentery and hanging lesser and greater omentums. He has some sensation for the elimination processes but no control. His iliac crests and attachments are very sore. I soothingly release some of his countless energy cysts. I do extensive cranial pumping along with the rock and glide technique. After fifty minutes he has had enough, and it is time for his pain medication.

Three weeks later he arrives at my house, still pale and thin, but he can already lift himself out of the high truck and down into his wheelchair. He reports that he has about seventy percent feeling in his right leg and no feeling from his knee down on his left side. He tells me that he lasted fifteen seconds when he attempted to stand during physiotherapy. The next time he lasted as long as the therapist asked him to stand.

This time I work on his feet and legs. During the whole-body evaluation, the dural tube seems too sensitive for traction, so I just do the rock and glide. His legs and feet lack vitality and motivation, so I do the rock and glide on them to essentially amp up the rhythm. I again work on energy cysts. Diaphragm releases on his knees work surprisingly well. He says that the work I am doing on his feet feels really good on the right one, but he can't feel it on his left.

Ryan still has a lot of pain in his hips. This is little wonder, being that the bones have acted like a slingshot on his digestive tract. The left iliac crest feels like one huge energy cyst. It softens but certainly does not dissipate entirely. I do some of the cranium techniques with the time that is left. He leaves with the same determined attitude he arrived with. He is resolute that even if he doesn't ride broncs again, he will rope.

By the third treatment, I can do the complete 10-Step Protocol. His favorite is the cranial base release. I can now start working with facilitated segments.

Ryan's surgeon reports that he is doing remarkably well. He is getting stronger all the time. Three and a half months after his accident, he is able to ride a stationery bicycle. He also drives a half-ton pickup, which he gets in and out of himself.

I only hope for Ryan's continued recovery and to be a part of it. A famous bull rider, Tuff Hedeman, once explained the term "cowboy up" to me. It means that you carry on when you are injured or down, even when the prospect of doing whatever you're about to try is so bleak that the best you can hope for is to live through it. Ryan is the definition of that.

Judy Pszyk
Bonnyville, Alberta, Canada
CranioSacral Therapy Practitioner since 2000

Feet First

✾ I am a dental assistant who has worked with the same dentist for twenty-nine years. When I developed temporomandibular joint (TMJ) disorder, I was referred to a specialist who deals with TMJ. He recommended that I wear a bruxism (grinding) night splint. After three such appliances, the TMJ persisted.

I knew that our town, though small (five thousand people), had a CranioSacral Therapist named Noreen. The specialist I saw had been referring his patients to her. I considered seeing her but just never seemed to have the time to call and book an appointment. The fact that I knew nothing about CranioSacral Therapy (CST) added to the delay.

Then a co-worker who was scheduled to see Noreen for whiplash problems mentioned that she would be unable to keep her appointment. I saw the opportunity to go myself, and so I took her time slot. I had no idea what to expect.

Noreen is also a registered massage therapist, so I assumed that CranioSacral Therapy would be similar to a massage. When I arrived at the appointment, Noreen asked me a few questions, made some chart notes, then instructed me to lie on her table. I thought this was okay, as she didn't ask me to remove any clothing. I assumed she would be working on my head and neck area.

She placed a heating pad across my chest area and a blanket over top. I was quite warm, but not totally relaxed, and I still had no idea what she was going to do. Then to my amazement she placed her hands on my feet. I lay there thinking, "I'm here for my jaw joint disorder—why is she touching my feet?" She then moved to my lower back (sacral area).

At this point I had to ask what she was doing. Noreen explained how the body is linked together. I admit I wasn't listening to most of what she said, because I was busy trying to anticipate her next move.

At the end of my hour-long appointment, I was not sure what I had just been through. She asked me how I was. I didn't really feel any different. She explained that, because of my chronic TMJ disorder of approximately twenty-five years, I would need more appointments.

I was very skeptical at this time that CST was right for me, but I thought I'd give it another try. After several appointments, I did get relief in my TMJ, neck, and shoulders. I stopped wearing my appliance. Some twenty sessions later, I felt I was cured!

I told my employer about Noreen, and we now regularly refer patients to her and rarely suggest splint therapy for TMJ disorder.

Noreen has helped me tremendously, and I truly trust her ability, abundant knowledge, and sense of humor. She tells me that I am a challenge! I am now seeing her for a sore hip and have the confidence she can help this too. I am no longer skeptical of her abilities as a CranioSacral Therapist, even though she starts with my feet!

Story by Corlys Gougeon
Submitted by Noreen Sparrow, RMT
Parry Sound, Ontario, Canada
CranioSacral Therapy Practitioner since 1992

Overnight Sensation

Several months ago one of my very elderly clients fell forward up a flight of stairs, hit her forehead, and then bounced down on her nose and chin. She had other injuries to her upper and lower extremities, as well as to each area that hit the edge of the stairs as she descended. Of course she was disoriented and quite confused.

A few hours after the fall she was transported to my office. She was deep purple-black over most of her face, and her nose and chin had been cut and were oozing and bandaged. Each area that had hit a stair was heavily bruised.

Because of all that my client had been through that day, I decided to apply the gentle techniques of CranioSacral Therapy (CST). I then asked her to return the next day so that I could follow up with traditional chiropractic.

Years previously, CST had helped me overcome a traumatic brain injury, so I knew how powerful the technique was. Yet I was unprepared for what I saw when I walked in that room the next day.

I thought I was going to see a badly bruised woman with possible shaken-brain syndrome and whiplash. Instead, I saw the lively, pink-faced, smiling woman I knew. She thought the rapid changes were normal for my care. I was astounded not only at the rapid changes, but also at the lack of symptoms that a fall like hers would generate.

I had spent seventeen years working with high-performance athletes and had taught at many national and world-class sports training centers throughout the world. After seeing the power of CST in this case, I decided to close my large practice and move to a smaller location with lower overhead and no employees so that I could offer one-hour CranioSacral Therapy sessions.

Khelly Webb, DC, CCSP, FIACA, CVCP
Long Beach, California
CranioSacral Therapy Practitioner since 2003

Anne's Story

After I finished taking CranioSacral Therapy, I wanted to use the technique on everyone. Friends, neighbors, and family were invited to try a session so that I could practice. Basically any client who showed even a remote interest in the therapy ended up on my table and was assessed for quality, amplitude, rhythm, and symmetry.

Anne, my sister, was one of these people. She would always get off the table and say, "I feel like a million bucks." After I took Cranio-Sacral Therapy, level two, she was the first one to ask me if she could stop by and check out what I had learned.

This time around I was able to tune in more. In doing so I discovered an energy disturbance. My hands were drawn to her thoracic region. As soon as I began the diaphragm release, her head started to roll slowly to one side, then pause, strain, and roll back to the other side. This kept repeating.

The image of a child's toy came to my mind—one of those round, hand-held games with three or more little metal balls that you try to get into the punched-out holes. If you tilt the game too far the balls already in their holes fall out again. So by the time you're down to the last ball, your movement is slow as you work with intent to help it find its place.

I took Anne's head in my hands and slowly followed the movement to the right side, where I offered a slight resistance. Her head went into extension to the point where she was facing me. A powerful pull of the dura held her so that she was literally resting with the top of her head against the table. "Are you OK?" I said, getting a little concerned. This was the first time I had witnessed such a strong response.

"Never felt better," she said with a grin. "Just didn't think it went back that far."

Suddenly the release came and her head straightened out then rolled to the left. At the end I again offered resistance. This time her head flexed onto her chest, and I could feel how her body was pulled up into a sitting position. I had to scramble around the corner of the table so that I didn't lose contact with her occiput. "What have you been eating?" Anne said. "I didn't think you would be able to push me around like a rag doll."

"That wasn't my doing," I said. "I could barely get around the corner of the table fast enough." Again I checked in with her to see if she was all right, and she said she was.

"I thought for a moment you were pushing me, because my body just came up like that. I can't even do it that smoothly when I'm doing my abdominal work. Oh, here we go again," Anne said. Her arms stretched out and came to rest between her legs, and her head nearly touched her knees. "I don't think I can bend any further," she said. No sooner had she finished saying that, but she went down further. "I think I'm going to kiss my butt," she said in a muffled voice, her head between her knees.

At that point I broke into laughter. We both laughed as she came out of the flexed position, tilted slightly toward me, and slowly stretched out on the table. My right hand moved down her spine in order to guide her into a recumbent position. She giggled and quipped, saying, "I couldn't do that again if you paid me. It's funny, while I'm doing all this I can still talk and laugh, and it doesn't seem to affect this process at all. It's as if I'm watching myself from outside my body."

My right hand was at the level of her eighth and ninth ribs, and my left hand was over her solar plexus. Her back began to arch higher and higher. "Oh brother," she said, groaning. "You're going to see if I can reach my butt this way too?" I couldn't help smiling. That turned to immediate concern, however, when a tremendous strain produced a loud crack from the area of the spine where I had my right hand.

"Did you hear that?" Anne said.

Yes, I heard that! I didn't want to show her that it had frightened me somewhat, though, and so I said out loud, "That was quite a release there, but you need not be alarmed. Your body will never take you anywhere you are not ready to go, and it will never inflict any harm on itself."

"I wasn't worried," she said. "But ever since I had that accident with the van five years ago, I've had a pain in that spot. Not really painful all the time, but it always aches, whether I'm standing up or lying down. I think it's gone now. It feels really good, open some-how."

Her body settled into a relaxed-breathing rhythm. I induced a still point and waited for her to sit up. She stretched, rolled her shoulders, and twisted her back in all directions.

"Yep, I think it's gone, but I'll let you know if it comes back," she said with a grin. We chatted some more and she moved her shoulders and back through all sorts of positions to see if she could find the discomfort, but it was truly gone.

Over a year has passed since that evening. Anne has enrolled in a massage therapy school and has taken a CranioSacral Therapy class. When she was told by her massage therapy instructors that she would be better off taking the CST course after she finished school, her response was: "That's the reason I'm here in the first place. Nothing can keep me from taking that course."

Anita Snippe, LMT
Manotick, Ontario, Canada
CranioSacral Therapy Practitioner since 2002

"I Don't Know How It Works; I Just Know It Does"

✿ Twenty years ago, I developed a severe infection following an emergency C-section. The infection traveled to many places, including my brain. I spent two months in the hospital, unable to care for my precious newborn. Family members feared for my life. Fortunately, my health improved, thanks to a lot of help from loving family and friends and inspiration from my daughter.

Two years later, though, I still had a walking disability. I just couldn't catch my balance. Doctors explained that parts of my brain were dead and that I was lucky to be alive. One even told me I'd never improve. He was a real source of inspiration to me—to prove him wrong! I have a stubborn streak, and I knew I was still improving and he wasn't going to stop me!

Flash forward about seventeen years. I regularly babysat for a friend whose son was seeing a physical therapist. She was really impressed with the therapist's gentle yet effective touch, as well as with her knowledge and willingness to speak in terms that my friend could understand without having a medical degree.

I was interested in what this miracle therapist, Alice Duddy, was doing. Then one day my friend told me that Alice thought she might be able to help me, too. I felt myself tune in, yet I also felt my protective instincts reminding me not to get my hopes up. It had been nineteen years. What could anyone do now?

I took Alice's name and number and told myself to set up an appointment when I had the time and mindset to handle the disappointment if another try was ineffective. Time went by, and I didn't call.

One day while I was babysitting, Alice came by the house to give therapy to my friend's little boy. She stroked his head. He fiddled with little toys she gave him. And I was amazed. He made no effort to leave her, and it seemed that she wasn't doing anything at all restrictive. I thought I could use that kind of massage just to have some time to relax!

As Alice explained to me what she was doing, I became more and more interested for myself, which is a fairly unusual phenomenon. I asked her a question about what I was experiencing. She continued working on him with those gentle hands while she talked to me about possibilities. I decided to give it a try.

A short time later, I went to her office. I'd seen her work, so I knew there was no pain involved, no condescending attitude about a miracle cure, no sugarcoated answers—none of the stuff I'd experienced so many times before. Yet here I was, a combination of nerves and high hopes all fluttering around inside me. I felt like a teenager heading for my first driving lesson. This was gonna be good, right? I kept telling myself to calm down, to not expect too much, to stay grounded.

Alice showed me to her little room. She massaged my head as we talked. I explained some of the problems I had, and she asked related questions. I kept thinking, "This is so easy." She did some gentle tugging on my ears and we talked about how different each ear felt to me. She softly felt different areas on my head. I thought she was just investigating; there could be no effect yet.

Then I sat up. Everything in my head felt different. I caught my breath and leaned back down. Alice assured me that I didn't need to hurry. She said it might take a little while for me to feel "normal," but I'd be fine. Nothing hurt, it just felt so different that I couldn't believe it.

For nineteen years I'd stayed near walls at home in case I needed them for support. Outside, I would hold onto my husband or, if alone, push a collapsible cart to hold my purse and provide me with balance. I would joke about walking like a drunk. I feared falling any time I didn't have something to hold onto.

My brain felt as if it were waking up after a very long sleep. Parts tingled. I hadn't experienced this feeling in over a decade.

Now I can walk through my home without holding onto anything. Sometimes I can even walk outside without holding things. Progress is usually steady, and every once in a while dramatic.

I remember calling Alice in tears because I'd just walked through a parking lot, up a curb, and into a store without holding onto my husband at all. I remember counting the seconds that I could stand on one foot before I lost my balance. I remember the utter amazement the first time I had the energy and ability to clean the kitchen and wash dishes after everyone had left a family party. Usually I had to sit down and tell everyone where to put things for me to work on the next day. My energy level and balance have drastically improved, and they are still improving!

I know that nineteen years of protecting myself against falling is making it hard for me to believe I can do some things. But Alice quietly works and reinforces any positive thoughts I have and never pushes me too quickly.

Alice and I have been working together for about a year now. Sometimes when I talk to others about it, I think that a year sounds like a long time. But then I remember that my brain was "dead" and is coming alive. That's huge work, and I need the time to adjust.

I don't understand the science of this gentle touch—I just know it works. I used to wear out pretty early in the day, and now I'm providing full-time foster care for a two-year-old! Alice Duddy has been a miracle worker in my life and I couldn't be more thankful!

Story by Cindi Bockweg, client
Submitted by Alice Duddy, PT
Framingham, Massachusetts
CranioSacral Therapy Practitioner since 1997

Liberated from Polio's Effects

A fifty-two-year-old woman suffering the effects of polio came to see me. She had to walk on her tiptoes on one foot to compensate for the shorter leg. She had endured numerous surgeries throughout her life to try to lengthen the leg—and she had the scars on her calf and Achilles to prove it.

At the time I began the CranioSacral Therapy (CST) session, I knew only that she had had polio, but I did not have the specifics. Her sphenoid was very compressed, and it felt like her face was sucked inward. The tissue began to soften. I detected the rhythm and felt the parietal bones spread. As I did a pelvic diaphragm release, her entire pelvis began to rotate out, as did her spine all the way up the diaphragms. It felt like a rope that was untwisting. I was drawn to do a regional tissue release on her right leg. I worked that for about twenty minutes.

I felt tissue releasing and her leg lengthening! I had goose bumps from my head to my toes but continued to allow her body to organize all the while. She was in a state of deep alpha and felt nothing, she said later. I felt so much movement. Then I began to work on her foot, and it also twisted and straightened!

After the session, she stretched and was very relaxed. She said she felt nothing physical, only deep relaxation like she had never felt before. When she got off the table, she began walking quickly back and forth. She was nearly hysterical with excitement. "I have never been able to do this in all my life!" she kept saying. When I realized what she was so ecstatic over, I was taken with emotion also. She was walking heel-to-toe with both feet! Not on her tiptoes.

She was in shock for about half an hour and continued her fast pacing back and forth in the office. That large shoe lift she always wore would no longer be needed.

I don't ever discount the miracles of CranioSacral Therapy. I reminded my patient of the potential the body has to heal itself when given the correct modalities. In about an hour's time, CST had accomplished what doctors had tried to achieve all of this woman's life.

Karen McGill, ND, BSNH, Herbalist
New Buffalo, Michigan
CranioSacral Therapy Practitioner since 2003

Old Injury Linked to Recurring Pneumonia

In 1987 I underwent abdominal surgery. Six weeks later I returned to my job as a physical therapist at a local hospital. I worked with respiratory in-patients and came across a lot of very ill people. Within a short time I contracted a severe respiratory infection that developed into left upper-lobe pneumonia.

Over the next twelve years I had many relapses, and probably contracted this same pneumonia on average twice per year, never less than once per year. I would be too ill to get out of bed, sometimes for one or two days, sometimes for a week. I was short of breath and coughed up thick, tenacious, dark-green sputum. It was cultured in the lab and revealed no growth of any identifiable infection, but I say anything that color had to be growing an army! It was doubtless a viral infection that I would always have to deal with.

I would get this pneumonia at times of stress, particularly work- or family-related. It would wipe me out. I began to feel old beyond my thirty-five years and developed a sense of despair. It felt like no matter how healthy a lifestyle I lived, no matter how well I ate and how much I exercised, I was truly helpless. I couldn't roughhouse with my small children or take my dog for a walk for several weeks out of each year. I saw myself as a respiratory cripple who would probably be buried by age fifty at the rate I was going.

Eventually, after almost twelve years of this nonsense, I asked to see a respirologist. I told him all my symptoms. I told him that I always knew when this pneumonia was going to happen, but there was nothing I could do about it. It would start with a cold, then progress down to the anterior portion of the left upper lobe, an area the size of a golf ball. When it was imminent, the area would tingle and effervesce. The feeling was subtle but unmistakable.

The look he gave me said it all. He told me that it was impossible to feel what I felt. His response felt cold and sneering, and I knew I had lost credibility with him as a therapist. How many others have endured the humiliation of being told by a physician that what they feel is not what they feel? And here I was with a healthcare background and knowledge of anatomy and physiology. He offered me a bronchoscopy, saying that what I had might be operable. I said I'd think about it.

It was in 1999 that I was drawn strongly to take a CranioSacral Therapy course. I had heard about the courses and was intrigued, yet intimidated by the syllabus. I knew there was an element of the esoteric involved, and it required an open mind. My right brain had been in hibernation for a lot of years but was beginning to come alive.

It seemed that everywhere I went I noticed something related to CranioSacral Therapy or The Upledger Institute. I had already explored emotional process work and was curious about Somato-Emotional Release. Then my cousin, a chef in Scotland, phoned me. He had just returned from catering an Advanced CranioSacral Therapy course in rural Scotland and was absolutely fascinated by what he had seen.

"That's enough!" I said to myself. "Time to take a course." Before I did, however, I first wanted to experience this modality. I asked a practitioner to give me a basic treatment, paying particular attention to my sore sacroiliac joint. I wasn't even thinking about my lungs.

The CranioSacral Therapist did what I learned later to be a basic 10-Step Protocol. As she went across my chest she was drawn to my left clavicular area. Her hands shook, the area pulsed and released heat, and I intuitively knew that I would never again have pneumonia. Nothing was said and, at the time, I had absolutely no idea what just happened. It turned out she had released a huge energy cyst caused by a fall on my knee years earlier, which had jammed my S.I. joint.

That was the autumn of 1999. Now, almost five years later, I have had no further hint of shortness of breath or pneumonia, and not one more sick day from work.

Needless to say, I now use CranioSacral Therapy as a huge part of my physical therapy practice. And anytime a client says, "You probably think this sounds crazy, but this is what I feel," I listen!

Heather Hodge, PT
Courtenay, British Columbia, Canada
CranioSacral Therapy Practitioner since 2000

A Friend Indeed

❀ Until I studied CranioSacral Therapy, I had never come across a healing modality that did so much with so little. One of my first incredible experiences was with a friend who is now a client.

She had been complaining of unusually severe migraine headaches. On several occasions she ended up being admitted to the hospital for a shot of Demerol. Along with the headaches, she would get a soft spot that felt like jelly near her front fontanelle, although she was over thirty-five years old. She also had numbing and tingling in her left arm, which quite often resulted in the swelling of her hand. This was attributed to a disc that "went out" every now and again. She had gone for physiotherapy, which had helped at the time; the problem still came back frequently to haunt her, however.

I managed to get her permission to treat her with CranioSacral Therapy. She was hesitant because she did not like to be touched and was very tense. I reassured her by saying that I would stop immediately if she was uncomfortable at any time.

At first evaluation, I found her rhythm to be quite erratic. I gently worked on the diaphragms and kept checking in with her about the touch to see if she was all right. Her body eventually started to relax and she began to feel at ease. I then treated her on another day to get her used to the feel of being treated. It was on her third visit that things really opened up for her.

When I greeted her that day she had very low energy and felt one of her migraines coming on. She was preparing for the worst, thinking that she might have to go to the hospital, which was the usual process. She was squinting due to the sensitivity of her eyes. Her arm was also numb and swollen.

I began to free up her frontal bones, which were stuck. Almost instantly, she felt an easing in the pressure of her headache. I continued with freeing up the other cranial bones.

I then got a strong sense to release the disc in her thoracic region. I followed and moved gently into place. My friend then said that she could feel the headache from her disc. It was a line up her spine and into the head. I asked if she was in pain, and she replied that it was uncomfortable but bearable.

Not long after that she said, "Oh, it's gone. It's fine now. No pain or discomfort." I asked if it was all right to stay there a while longer. She said that would be fine and to keep doing whatever I was doing because something was working.

I continued to follow the tissue, offering energy when needed. After what seemed like only five minutes, but in reality was close to fifteen, a movement happened within her spine. She said, "Oh my God, did you feel that?" I replied that I had and asked how the pain in her head was. When she answered, "What pain?" I knew that we were on the right track.

When the session was finished for the day, I asked how she felt. She told me that she was tired but not in pain and that she actually felt very good. Just before she was ready to leave, I noted that she was now very talkative and bubbly. She was smiling and cracking jokes.

I later got an e-mail from her titled "Your Magic Hands!" The first sentence read as follows: "I can't even begin to tell you how wonderful I feel thanks to you. I could cry I am so happy about it. Thanks again and again and again!"

I now treat my friend if she feels a headache coming on, which is rarely. She feels too good at any other time to book a treatment.

Wendy Morley
London, Ontario, Canada
CranioSacral Therapy Practitioner since 2001

Deep Sleep at Last

Shortly after my first CranioSacral Therapy workshop I was practicing on as many clients as I could. My fifth person was a frail, fifty-four-year-old woman with chronic obstructive pulmonary disease (COPD) and the beginning stages of emphysema. She carried a small oxygen bottle in case she needed it. The client indicated that she never got more than two hours of sleep at a clip.

I was eager to practice the 10-Step Protocol and see what CranioSacral Therapy was all about. I was quickly to become a firm believer.

The next day this woman called to inform me that she had slept twelve straight hours! The excitement and happiness in her voice was reward in itself. She felt the positive effects for about three days before the old symptoms returned. Needless to say, she wanted more treatments. This is a powerful therapy, and I thank Dr. John Upledger for sharing it with me.

Ray Turner, PhD, LMT
Amityville, New York
CranioSacral Therapy Practitioner since 2004

The Underlying Current

❁ The first time I felt the craniosacral system fluid I was hooked. The tissues, muscles, bones, and all aspects of the body came alive as it moved, stopped, twisted, turned, unwound, and released.

My clients never know what they will be experiencing with each session as I help to guide them through their bodies. They are amazed at how quickly, easily, and gently their bodies heal.

One such woman came to see me because she was experiencing excruciating pain in her right side and breast that no drug could even touch.

In the first session I used a combination of CranioSacral Therapy and lymphatic drainage, letting my hands follow the pathways to release the toxins and restrictions. This woman could barely handle any light touch because the pain was so severe. Within the first session I was able to touch her without causing pain; this allowed me to go deeper.

On the second visit the woman said she was still in pain, but the results since the last time were evident. During this session I was able to get deeper and release the lung area, which helped her to breathe better.

The third visit I was at last able to work with the liver, which was hard and painful to the touch. The first two visits did not allow for this, as I needed to clean up the surrounding areas first so the liver could be freed.

I used less than the weight of a nickel to begin working with the liver. As the rhythms and fluids started to ease and change, the pain shifted to the back and then to the front, where the fluid was able to release through the thoracic duct.

We also used SomatoEmotional Release to help her get past resentment in her life. She discovered a whole new world in releasing the rage that had been pent up in her for so long. This was done gently and compassionately. The drama and trauma did not have to be relived.

The woman breathed a sigh of relief. She could actually touch her right side without wincing.

Next I attended to the rib under her breast, which was extremely sore to the touch. I placed my hands on the areas to which I was directed by the body, and I felt the familiar movement of the cerebrospinal fluid. The bone wiggled and torqued gently under my touch. I could feel the bone as it seemed to sigh and let go. Instead of feeling dense and stuck, it was now alive and free. Once again the woman felt greatly improved as she moved that area of her body.

The smile on the woman's face was incredulous, though she still feared the worst from this pain. But at last she felt hope that she would be rid of this terrible problem. I feel so blessed to be able to assist people so gently through the fluids and tissues of their bodies.

I marvel every day at how quickly people are relieved of stress, emotions, and pain through CranioSacral Therapy. They leave my office smiling, full of hope and newfound happiness that there is another way. Even if they don't understand how this happened, I know a great service has been done by the gentle placement of my hands.

I love the movement within the body and sense it on every level. The bonus is that I see ongoing results within my practice. This is why I love this work. Each day I learn more. I am fascinated by how powerful and profound the healing process of the body can be when we are ready to explore its full potential.

Susan Faber, CBI
Cochrane, Alberta, Canada
CranioSacral Therapy Practitioner since 1999

A New Life and a New Career

❀ My story involves a twenty-nine-year-old mother of two. She discovered CranioSacral Therapy by chance after searching out every therapy she could possibly find to help with severe and unrelenting trigeminal neuralgia to the left side of her face and head.

The woman's symptoms had begun slowly, with frequent headaches, after she had all her wisdom teeth pulled. Within six months the problem developed into a nightmare. She tried everything from acupuncture and massage therapy to various doctors and dentists, all of which only seemed to aggravate the problem. She was unable to work and was, at times, barely coping from hour to hour.

It wasn't until the woman's acupuncturist tried some "cranial work" that she finally had some minor relief. This was nearly a year after the original surgery, and by now she was also suffering from depression and anxiety due to the pain, and had lost a considerable amount of weight.

The acupuncturist didn't speak a lot of English, so when her client began to ask questions about the therapy, she gave the woman a CranioSacral Therapy (CST) textbook. This opened a whole new world for the woman. The idea of the bones in her head still moving as an adult, and possibly being restricted, was exactly what she had been feeling.

The woman lived in a rural area where it was difficult to find therapists, so she went on the Internet and signed up for a Cranio-Sacral Therapy class in Vancouver in the spring of 2003. By the end of the four-day course, she was amazed not only by the concepts of the therapy, but by the fact that she went home relieved of her depression and in considerably less pain. She continued to seek out therapists in her area and immediately signed up to take the next CST course.

Not only did CranioSacral Therapy give this woman back her

life, it also gave her a new and very rewarding career. I know this because I am that woman, and I am so very thankful to have found CranioSacral Therapy. It has changed my life in so many ways, and I know that having lived through this painful experience helps me immensely in my practice.

I am only just beginning my journey as a CranioSacral Therapist, but I have already had some amazing results with my clients. I love to share what I know with people and to help them find their path to healing.

It has been two years now since that fateful surgery on my wisdom teeth. I still have some minor discomfort, but I believe that in time I will be completely healed. In the meantime I am enjoying the chance to share this amazing therapy with the world.

Kjara Brecknell
Salmon Arm, British Columbia, Canada
CranioSacral Therapy Practitioner since 2003

Concussions, Snowballs, and Volleyball

Richard was a twenty-three-year-old college student who arrived at the clinic for assessment and treatment of his headaches. He had been a competitive athlete from a young age, playing sports such as rugby in high school and, most recently, varsity volleyball.

Richard's problems began at the age of thirteen, when he was knocked out during a rugby tackle and remained unconscious for seven minutes. Since that time he had been concussed on ten additional occasions. Most of them were sports-related. The last time he was knocked out was because a random snowball hit him. That incident occurred a year prior to his initial visit with me. Forced to give up playing volleyball, he was now acting as coach, although his goal was to play again.

Richard's primary complaint was daily headaches that had plagued him for the last two years. He had been checked out by neurologists and thoroughly investigated with both a CT and MRI scan, but no one could provide him any answers. The only recommendation was to take Advil (an anti-inflammatory) when required for the pain. As a twenty-three-year-old fit man, he did not wish to be on painkillers for the rest of his life.

Initially Richard was assessed by a colleague of mine who focused her efforts on treating some stiffness in his neck with traditional manual therapy. Seeing no change in his symptoms, she suggested that he see me, as she was aware that I did "that craniosacral stuff."

When I first saw Richard, he had no idea what CranioSacral Therapy was, but he was game to try any therapy to get some relief. I assessed him and realized immediately that the amplitude of his craniosacral rhythm was significantly decreased on his left, and that his left temporal bone was not rotating as it should with each cycle. I questioned him about some of his head injuries, and he reported that several of the knocks, including the hit with the snowball, had been to his left temple. I performed the 10-Step Protocol that day, and he went on his way.

The following week, Richard reported that his concentration level for his studying had significantly improved; his head felt less "foggy." While his headaches were still occurring, they had less intensity. I saw him for a total of six treatments, each time performing techniques from the 10-Step Protocol to improve and balance his craniosacral rhythm.

By the last two visits, Richard's headaches had subsided completely. He told me that he finally realized they were gone when he was talking to his mother on the phone and she said, "How is your headache?" He had to think about it for a second before replying, "Wait a minute, I don't have a headache!"

At our second-to-last session, I advised Richard that he could begin to return to a light training regime to see how his body coped with the increased demand on it. When I saw him the following week, he had played in a volleyball tournament (instead of coaching) and was happy to report that he was still symptom-free. When I told him he had just made my day, he replied, "You've made my life!"

Richard's story illustrates so clearly how CranioSacral Therapy can help someone dramatically in just a few sessions. This young man was able to participate again in the sports he enjoys and will hopefully stay out of the way of snowball fights!

Nancy J. Fletcher, RPT
Calgary, Alberta, Canada
CranioSacral Therapy Practitioner since 2002

Slow but Steady Progress

❁ Thirty-four-year-old Eric was referred to me by two physical therapists employed at a nearby hospital. They were allowed to do only minimal CranioSacral Therapy, and when Eric's insurance no longer covered his treatment, he was referred to me.

Seventeen years prior, Eric had undergone jaw surgery that went awry. He went into cardiac arrest and was in a coma for seven days. He lost his vision and his ability to move.

Since that time Eric had regained his vision and relearned how to move. He still had impaired fine-motor skills, poor balance, a damaged gait, mobility problems, and vision and speech impediments. Despite these challenges, Eric had a college degree in communication. He lived independently with his dog, was employed, and was very physically active. He rode a recumbent tricycle, swam, and did weight training. His outlook on life was very positive and upbeat.

Our initial session revealed jammed temporals, parietals, and frontalis. The atlanto-occipital joint was very stuck. From the top of the dural tube, muscle activity along with releasing and relaxing of tissue could be detected in his legs, pelvic girdle, shoulder girdle, and arms. After the session, relaxation in these areas remained for several days, and he slept better.

Since March 2004 we have worked on a schedule of weekly hour-long sessions. Each week sees a little progress. He is standing taller; the scapulae are more level; and his rib cage is more equilateral. His face is beginning to change as well. His quick grin is more even and central to his face.

Eric is very proactive in his treatments. He continues weight training and other physical activities. Once a month he receives a massage and a chiropractic adjustment. The chiropractor has commented that the adjustments have become easier since Eric began the CranioSacral Therapy.

Each day for ten to fifteen minutes, Eric lies on tennis balls for still point induction. He has had remarkable experiences using these. He has begun to feel muscle sensation—the nerve synapses firing and tingling throughout his torso. Over the weeks, these new sensations have begun to move into his extremities, the pelvic girdle, and down his spine. Some of the sensations have become permanent.

Since Eric experiences such great success with the tennis balls, I have him lie on them during treatment. Employing them seems to help his body move through the stuck areas more quickly.

I frequently V-spread stubborn or hard-to-reach areas. If I V-spread the diaphragm with the ilia, for example, the entire pelvic girdle will shift. The diaphragm V-spread with L5 [lumbar vertebra] is another powerful release area for Eric.

In our last two sessions I have begun work in his mouth. Already there is a noticeable change in his speech, and his jaw is more aligned. The vomer, however, remains stuck. Eric reports a lot of sensation and activity in his head. Recently he lay on the tennis balls and the vomer shifted a bit. It seems there are a lot of challenges to be met inside his mouth.

Eric and his personal trainer Steve shared their respective observations with me:

Eric: The main thing I have noticed is that my back spasms have greatly decreased. A slight tightness still occurs periodically, but the entire debilitating episodes have all but disappeared. Also, my hands, neck, and shoulders seem to be generally looser on a day-to-day basis. After a weight-training session my muscles seem to not tighten up to a painful degree as they used to, and the recovery time has decreased. To a lesser degree, I am starting to become more in tune with my body (e.g. postural and mobility corrections).

Steve: The main benefit I see from the therapy is that Eric is more fluid in his everyday movements (e.g. walking, standing, getting up from a sitting position). I also notice that Eric seems to have far fewer painful muscle spasms, and his tone has decreased significantly. Immediately after a session, Eric's posture is great, but it gradually decreases as the hours and days pass. It is improving, however, to the point that he stays completely upright for up to three days after a session. The secondary benefit I see is that Eric seems to be in a better place mentally since starting these sessions.

Ellie Brown Gee, CST
Pawcatuck, Connecticut
CranioSacral Therapy Practitioner since 1989

No More Dizzy Spells

❁ Several months ago I was spending the evening with some friends when all of a sudden I was overwhelmed with dizziness. After an hour or so of this, my friends decided they should take me to the hospital.

After many tests I was diagnosed with vertigo by the emergency room doctor. He gave me a prescription to help with the dizzy spells. The medicine helped some, but the dizziness continued. Most episodes lasted at least an hour, and some of them caused me to be extremely nauseous.

I had been going to Jasuti Goss for massage therapy. When I told her about my dizzy spells, she recommended that I try CranioSacral Therapy (CST). She told me about another client whom she had successfully treated for vertigo several months earlier. I didn't understand how this therapy worked, but I figured I had nothing to lose, so I agreed to try CST.

Nothing much seemed to be happening in the first few sessions. Jasuti explained that it might take a series of treatments and encouraged me to continue. I think it was after the fourth session that I realized I was not having any more dizzy spells. I had suffered with this horrible dizziness for months and, to my surprise, after just a few CranioSacral Therapy sessions they had completely ended.

It has now been a few months since the original series of CST, and I still have had no dizzy spells. I recently began to feel like the dizziness might be trying to start up again, so I went to Jasuti for another treatment. So far, so good! I haven't had another dizzy spell.

I still don't understand how CranioSacral Therapy works. What I do know is that it works, and that is all I care about. I am very grateful for both Jasuti and CranioSacral Therapy!

Story by Leona Loucks
Submitted by Jasuti Goss, NCMT
Anderson, Indiana
CranioSacral Therapy Practitioner since 1998

Resetting Randi

✿ Think about this next time you watch someone in a wheelchair deftly negotiate a busy shopping mall corridor: It may have taken this person up to two hours to get out of bed that morning, go to the bathroom, and put on some clothes. Those legs, which look peaceful and still in that wheelchair, move with ferocious independence when their owner awakens and tries to get through the daily routine we take for granted. This is a case of severe muscle spasticity. This has been Randi's life for nearly two years.

Spasticity is a common condition for individuals with spinal cord injury. It varies from mild muscle stiffness to severe, uncontrollable leg movements. It occurs when communication flow between the spinal cord and brain is interrupted.

Randi is a former professional motorcycle drag racer. She was injured in August 2002 at the completion of a quarter-mile race in which she made a crucial error and hit the pavement as a human projectile at ninety miles per hour. Her vertebrae were shattered at T6 and T10 [thoracic vertebrae]. At T6, the two outer layers of her spinal cord were stretched and rebounded, resulting in her paralysis. She has no movement or feeling below the level of T12 [bottom of her rib cage].

Randi's legs seem to operate as a separate entity from the rest of her body, even though she takes medication to prevent them from twisting into a permanent pretzel. As long as she is in her wheelchair, her legs are calm; but any movement out of the chair, such as therapy, exercise, or using the bathroom, results in strong involuntary hip flexion and leg adduction, especially on the left side. The constant pull has given her an elevated left hip and scoliosis.

I met Randi in September 2003 when I was hired as the massage therapist at a training and fitness facility dedicated to neuromuscular recovery for individuals with spinal cord injuries.

The techniques I use with spinal cord-injured (SCI) clients are the same as those who are fully able-bodied, except the goals may be different. I usually employ a combination of Swedish massage, Positional Release trigger-point therapy, Myofascial Release, and CranioSacral Therapy.

I completed my first CranioSacral Therapy class in July 2002, while still in massage school. Since that time, I have incorporated phases of the 10-Step Protocol into nearly all of my massages, and I like to end sessions with the cranial holds.

Randi, like her SCI peers, enjoys deep massage on her upper trunk, since nearly all of her movement is concentrated there. Unless there are special issues, I massage affected limbs and other areas on both para- and tetraplegics. Randi shared with me that even though she can't feel me touching her below her injury, she *sees* me on her muscles, *knows* I'm working them, and internally relaxes. She had experienced massage before her accident, and her mind and body haven't forgotten how it affects her. She says, "I know that internally you are loosening fascia, like taking Silly Putty and molding it back into place."

Lying on her back tends to exacerbate Randi's spasms. During the first ten minutes of our sessions, her left hip usually flexes at intervals, like a slow, separate heartbeat, until she relaxes into the massage. Even after her hip is quiet, it remains slightly elevated off the table, with her left knee turned inward. If I touch any part of either leg, both legs will flex and her adductors tighten, placing her in a position resembling a child who is about to wet her pants.

At our third session, I introduced Randi to CranioSacral Therapy (CST), and her response was very positive. Her left hip and leg relaxed to the point of nearly lying flat on the table, and she enjoyed how she felt mentally afterward.

We did not do CST again until one month later, on a day when her legs were particularly uncooperative. Her trainer asked if I could work on her adductors, as they were extremely tight, and Randi asked if I could do CST again.

I proceeded through the 10-Step Protocol, feeling Randi's hip slowly drop under my hand during the pelvic diaphragm release. As I worked through the cranial holds, her breathing deepened, and I knew she was in a favorite place somewhere. Her legs lay flat.

While she was in this place, I walked to the side of the table and gently and slowly cradled her right leg, then lifted and abducted it enough to be able to work on her adductors. I waited for it to seize and remained alert to the possibility of her knee flying into my face. I was able to complete my work and then move to her more capricious left leg. To my surprise and delight, it allowed me to duplicate the motions I had achieved on her right leg.

I had seen and heard about the impact of CranioSacral Therapy from some of my other clients prior to this session, but this episode demonstrated the real power of CST and its almost magical effects. Needless to say, Randi was thrilled and relieved that her legs relaxed for at least an hour, and I was in awe of the experience.

Randi later told me that when we do CST, "It feels like you're resetting my spinal column, like you're pushing my reset button."

For several months after that session, we were unable to duplicate that amazing encounter. Though I work on her almost weekly, we don't do CST every time, as she often desires deep massage on her back and shoulders while prone. Oddly enough, however, during the course of writing this story Randi requested CST and we managed to trick her legs into allowing me to hold them and massage her adductors again. Happily, both of our reset buttons were pushed with the experience.

Cynthia Herman, LMT
Mason, Ohio
CranioSacral Therapy Practitioner since 2002

All I Want for Christmas Is My Energy

❀ Harry walked into my office one June afternoon. With great difficulty he made his way down the hall, stopping every few steps to catch his breath.

Harry had been born with one abdominal kidney, which had stopped functioning. With mortality staring him in the face, he was left with one option: a kidney transplant.

Wasting no time, the doctors at Cleveland Clinic found Harry's sister to be a perfect match, and the surgery was performed. Afterward, Harry's doctors pronounced him "doing as well as can be expected." This wasn't enough for Harry. Having been given a second chance at life, he was not satisfied with having just a functioning kidney. He wanted to go on trips with his family, take long walks with his sister, and conduct the county orchestra in its annual Christmas concert, as he had for many years.

Harry was exhausted all the time, which the doctors attributed to his dangerously low red-blood-cell count. For the year leading up to his visit with me, the doctors at Cleveland Clinic did everything to trigger a change, but Harry still could only walk a few slow steps before having to rest. His skin was pale, his muscle tone was poor, and Harry felt defeated.

Harry had only come to see me because his wife made the appointment for him. He could not begin to imagine what massage therapy could do for him in this serious condition. He was a good sport, though, and I found him very willing to listen as I tried to explain what my previous experiences had been, what we were trying to accomplish, what I was finding, and what changes I was hoping to see.

Harry had never heard of CranioSacral Therapy before his first session, but he would never forget it.

I had never felt a happy organ before this. Harry's new kidney resonated happily in his left iliac region. It just needed a little help to nestle into its new home. Once the trauma of the surgery was removed from the tissues, the kidney had become his own. The experience was much like picking up an upset infant and feeling him relax in your arms.

Harry felt every resonation, every movement. He could "feel his tissues crawling," as he put it, while my hands were following. He felt the releases of the injury from the surgery and how the area then relaxed. He was amazed and excited by his new experience, as he felt the heavy weight leaving his body.

We decided to have sessions twice a week. The swelling in Harry's abdomen and legs diminished; his color got better; and he felt more energetic. Soon he was walking the entire length of the hall without stopping.

Three weeks later, when Harry had his regular checkup at Cleveland Clinic, the doctors were amazed at his progress. His red-blood-cell count had improved enough that his appointment with the hematologist was canceled.

We had quite a few sessions throughout the year, and it was a pleasure to watch the weekly changes. Harry's improvement was great and continuous. He not only gained the energy he needed to practice with the orchestra, but he was able to conduct the Christmas concert.

He now plays golf a couple of times a week, travels, and takes pride in walking faster and having better stamina than his healthy buddies. I still see him on a monthly basis. These days, though, Harry schedules appointments not just for himself, but for his wife, too.

Ilona E. Trommler, LMT
Westlake, Ohio
CranioSacral Therapy Practitioner since 1998

On the Relief of Chronic Sinusitis

Jeff is a thirty-seven-year-old male who initially came to my office for help with old shoulder injuries (bilateral torn rotator cuffs) that he had refused to have surgery on some years prior. The visit had been a gift from his parent, who thought he would appreciate the stress-reduction benefit of CranioSacral Therapy (CST).

Amazed with the increased range of motion of his right shoulder after that one visit, he scheduled a second appointment the following week for the left shoulder. Once again he experienced substantial improvement in his range of motion and general relaxation. After that, he occasionally came by for a general CranioSacral Therapy tune-up.

Then, in the spring of 2003, Jeff called saying that he had very bad sinusitis and wanted to know if CST could help. When he arrived, I noted that the sinus areas around the eyes were extremely swollen and inflamed. He had no eyelid folds, and the eye openings were narrow secondary to the edema.

Jeff reported that he could never recall being without sinusitis symptoms. He had experienced two significant accidents when he was five years old. One was a fall against a concrete block in which he struck the left upper lip area. The second was when he was attending a baseball game with his father and was struck on the left upper lip and nose area. He suffered a broken nose that time and required seventeen sutures to the inner aspect of his left upper lip. He had had two sinus drainage surgeries from an excellent ENT specialist, with minimal relief, and was considering a third surgery prior to receiving CranioSacral Therapy.

In addressing the symptoms, I completed a brief, basic 10-Step Protocol and then focused on mobilization of the cranial bones. It was very obvious to both this client and me that the cranial bones in the left temporal area were completely immobile, while the right temporal bones moved quite well.

Due to Jeff's previous positive results with CranioSacral Therapy, he was extremely patient and cooperative during the three appointments it took to completely mobilize all of the impacted cranial bones.

Each session was dramatic. The first reduced the swelling of the eyes so much that his wife said to him when he got home, "Your eyes are bigger!" During the second session, the cranial bones began to move one by one. Then there was a loud click. "That's my teeth hitting together on the left side," he said. "They don't usually do that."

Over the next five days, large quantities of mucus drainage occurred. The entire shape of Jeff's face changed as the bones were mobilized. Symmetry was restored; TMJ symptoms were relieved; and sinusitis symptoms vanished with treatment.

I continue to see Jeff periodically for tune-up sessions or if he needs relief of a specific symptom. It has not been necessary to do additional cranial bone mobilization. He tells me that for many years he took daily doses of antihistamines and prescription medication to alleviate his sinusitis symptoms. He has not required this medication in more than a year now. Jeff credits CST for this and does not hesitate to tell family and friends of this change. He is a great example of the benefits possible with CranioSacral Therapy—even thirty years after an injury.

But the story doesn't end there. In February 2004, Jeff called early one Friday morning with an urgent request that I see his son Wade that afternoon. He had an important vocal audition scheduled the next day, and he had developed a cold with sinus congestion and coughing. The audition was for admission to the School of the Arts, and no make-up day was available for any candidate who could not perform his talent on the appointed day.

I provided almost two hours of CranioSacral Therapy to the boy that day. I focused on the eustachian tubes, ears, sinuses, neck, and upper chest. Although young, he was as cooperative as any adult upon whom I have worked. The results were excellent. There was drainage of mucus and elimination of the nasal vocal qualities that were initially so apparent.

Jeff reported the following week that the difference in his son's singing was remarkable. In April his son was notified of his acceptance to the School of the Arts.

In May, I made a house visit to give father and son a tune-up. Wade said, "I told my friends at school I was going to have a treatment by Jeannie. They asked, 'Is she really a genie?' I told them yes!"

Doing CranioSacral Therapy may not make you a genie, but on occasion you have very nice things happen.

Jean M. Reid, RNC, LMT
West Palm Beach, Florida
CranioSacral Therapy Practitioner since 2000

CST Makes Life Worth Living Again

✽ I received a call one day from a woman whose daughter had gotten my name from a therapist I went to school with. Her husband had been suffering from tinnitus for some time, ever since he'd had pneumonia, and nothing seemed to help his condition. His physicians said the next step would be "exploratory" surgery, and he did not want to go down that road. She wanted to know if CranioSacral Therapy could help.

I saw this client for the first time on January 6, 2004. I could sense that he was somewhat skeptical and was there because his wife wanted him to be. In fact, after our first session, he even admitted he was a skeptic, but he also said he had never experienced anything like that before. He rescheduled for one week later.

When he arrived, I asked him how he was doing. He reported that the ringing in his ears was about the same, but all the "bad feelings" associated with the ringing had lessened. For him, that was a major improvement. He didn't exactly know what I was doing, but if it continued to make him feel better, then he would continue to come back.

I saw this man pretty much on a weekly basis for about seven weeks. After that we agreed to try every other week and were eventually able to stretch his visits to every three weeks.

During this period, the number of times he needed to stop during the day to lie down on the floor to get some relief became less frequent. Our goal was to get him to a point where he would only need to come in for periodic tune-up.

While the ringing sensation is still present, this man's quality of life has improved tremendously. At the time of this writing, we are trying to schedule his visits on a monthly basis.

It has been very rewarding as a therapist to see not only the physical improvement in my client's life, but also his willingness to be open to other possibilities for his healing. The following is a direct quote from him:

"I cannot say enough about the therapy I have received from Judy. Before I came to her I was in agony. I had a loud ringing in my ears that was accompanied by dizziness, disorientation, and a run-down feeling.

"I was very skeptical about coming to see Judy, but it has turned into one of the most important things I have done in my life. Before, I had seen three different doctors; none of them provided any relief. After the last one, the only option I was given was exploratory surgery. I recommend Judy and the [CranioSacral Therapy] procedure to family members and friends. It has made life worth living again."

Judy Molique, LMT
Cincinnati, Ohio
CranioSacral Therapy Practitioner since 2000

Brain Damage, Autism, or Other?

✽ I began my CranioSacral Therapy career by giving my massage therapy clients complimentary demonstrations of what I had been learning. Within two months, ninety percent of them had converted to CranioSacral Therapy.

Susan came to see me after receiving a gift certificate from one of these CST converts. Upon completing the session, she asked if her twenty-five-year-old daughter Rebecca could come in the following day.

Rebecca had been the victim of shaken-baby syndrome at the age of four months. After the injury, she had changed from a smiling, cooing, happy baby to being unresponsive, lethargic, and drooling. As she grew, she was diagnosed as brain-damaged, with an IQ of 50.

The mother had dedicated the past twenty-five years to looking for and trying various recommended techniques to possibly improve her child's intellect and mental functioning. She had met with very little success. Additionally, as an adolescent and young adult, Rebecca had been subjected to abuse by some people in the name of education/training/development. She was fearful as a direct result of these abuses.

Susan always had a genuine goal of finding a means of treatment that would allow her daughter to eventually live independently and with minimal supervision. Rebecca was so limited and afraid of the environment outside her home due to her life experiences, she rarely ventured out to socialize. Her days consisted of working in a sheltered workshop, assigned to the traumatic brain injury unit, where she performed simple repetitive tasks. She went only back and forth to the workshop. Susan had remarried seven years prior but had never gone on a honeymoon or even taken a trip without her daughter also going.

Susan and Rebecca arrived the next day. We allowed the office door to remain slightly ajar so that Rebecca would not feel threatened. I also clearly gave her permission to move my hands or tell me to move my hands if anything I did was uncomfortable for her. She was able to tolerate an entire hour of basic protocol procedures without apparent fear or needing to move my hands. She readily agreed to return.

Subsequent visits, scheduled every other week, were relaxed and comfortable. Susan scheduled treatment for herself on the alternate weeks.

With just basic protocol measures, remarkable changes began to occur in Rebecca. She requested an analog watch so that she could learn to tell "real time." She began to spontaneously visit a special trusted neighbor more often. She made better grooming and style choices. And she was much more alert.

The sheltered workshop called six weeks after we began treatment to happily report that Rebecca stood up to a bully in her group twice that day by simply looking directly at him and refusing to do his work when he ordered her to do it. Previously she would not even make eye contact with aggressors, and would certainly never hold her own ground.

As she received inner-mouth work, Rebecca's TMJ symptoms were relieved, her asymmetrical face shape became symmetrical, and Mom excitedly noted, "Her eyes are the same size now!"

Rebecca's mood lifted and all aspects of her being became brighter. Mom reported that Rebecca had been promoted out of the TBI unit to work in a higher-functioning group at the sheltered workshop. When I complimented Rebecca on this, I speculated how rarely such a promotion must occur. She broadly smiled and joyously stated, "Jeannie, it never happens!"

We had begun all this work just after Christmas 2000. By July 4, 2001, Susan and her husband were able to take a long-overdue honeymoon, because Rebecca was able to stay with friends for the seven days they were gone.

Susan was so pleased with her daughter's progress that she began to study CranioSacral Therapy with The Upledger Institute and is now practicing CST in her community.

Rebecca continued to make amazing strides, and by summer of 2003 was able to move from her mom's home into a supervised-living group home. There she has responsibility for her own self-care, finances, and activities—the very things her mom worked toward and hoped could be achieved in Rebecca's life.

This work is my passion and a source of incredible joy to me. If this is as good as it gets, I am truly blessed and grateful.

Jean M. Reid, RNC, LMT
West Palm Beach, Florida
CranioSacral Therapy Practitioner since 2000

Pain and a Writer's Block

❁ Mrs. Flor is a writer and grandmother who came to me with a pain in her head on the right side behind her ear. She told me she had been suffering from this pain for more than fifteen years and that it never went away or gave her any rest.

She had been to numerous doctors and specialists, but none were able to resolve or improve the pain. She came to me at the recommendation of a friend who had told her about CranioSacral Therapy.

Feeling in a perpetual fog and extremely low on energy, Mrs. Flor was experiencing writer's block, which had rendered her unable to advance on the book she was writing. She no longer had energy to clean her house or work in her garden. She had low back pain and was resting all the time. She told me she felt uninspired and unable to go on like this.

In the first session I worked with her low back, neck, and head. I found her right temporal bone very restricted and felt a pulling at the cranial base. She told me she occasionally felt like she had lost her balance. I released a strong pulling through the tentorium by doing a release for both temporal bones. I also worked to free up the sutures between the temporals and occiput, as well as the parietal bones.

Mrs. Flor said that she was feeling relaxed as I got her up off the table. One week later she came back for her second appointment and informed me that everything was a little better. Her energy was coming back and her headaches were not as severe or as frequent.

As I worked with Mrs. Flor's cranium, I felt the right side was not quite as restricted as it had been the previous week. I spent the majority of an hour at her occiput, parietal, and temporal bones, the membranes surrounding and partitioning the brain, and at the fascia and muscles in her neck.

She also began telling me stories about her life, running the river and raising her family. Her husband had been in an accident years prior that left him disabled with back pain and unable to work. Again, when she got up off the table she told me that she felt better and very relaxed.

The next week Mrs. Flor came back for her appointment elated. Though still experiencing some light headaches and occasional dizziness, the majority of the pain in her head on the right side had not come back since our last treatment. After fifteen years it was gone! She was back to cleaning her house and working in the yard. Her energy was not a hundred percent, but it was much better, and she felt her inspiration returning for the book she was writing.

Mrs. Flor came back three weeks later for another treatment and gave me a copy of what she had written as a way to say thank you. She was very appreciative of how much better she was feeling. The pain never returned to the right side of her head. Her low back was much improved. She felt her neck was more comfortable and had better range of motion. Plus, the fog she was in completely lifted. Mrs. Flor continued to improve to the point that she didn't need to come anymore. She still enjoyed coming once a month, though, as a treat to herself.

Heather Navarrete-Linnemeyer, BA, LMT, CST-D
Grants Pass, Oregon
CranioSacral Therapy Practitioner since 1995

Continuity

✳ A few years ago I was contacted by a gentleman who was in town on a business trip. He had been receiving weekly CranioSacral Therapy (CST) in his hometown for about a year. His therapist recommended that he continue with this therapy during his trip. He was going to be in town two weeks.

I interviewed this man before his first visit with me. He described the nervous breakdown that had led him to begin CST in the first place. He had received electroshock therapy during his hospitalization as part of the treatment protocol. He had been unable to work after that—until he started CranioSacral Therapy, which he said had helped him unscramble his thought processes. This was his first business trip since his illness.

He was rather nervous when he arrived for his appointment, but became at ease after we visited and he got on the table. I used arcing to identify his heart/pericardium fascia as the priority area to treat for this session. The gentle CST touch prompted him to begin a SomatoEmotional Release. As he looked into his heart, he was reunited with an aspect of himself that he had separated from during his breakdown. Great calmness followed this reunion and remained with him for the duration of his visit.

I treated this client twice more and worked on rigidity in his left temporoparietal region, the temporomandibular joint area, and also inside his mouth. The left-side tissue tension, he said, was a lingering after-effect of the electroshock therapy; it was where the electrode had been placed.

At the conclusion of our third and final visit, the man reported that his left eye felt awake following completion of the intraoral cranial work. This was a very pleasant change for him.

I wrote a note detailing his visits with me to his CranioSacral Therapist. I received this reply: "Thank you for your note. What's funny is that we were planning on doing mouth work when he returned . . . great pickup."

As a therapist, I find it an interesting confirmation of Cranio-Sacral Therapy that the technique protocols, applied by two different therapists with different primary professional training (physical therapy and massage therapy), produced uninterrupted continuity of care for this client.

The cornerstone of CranioSacral Therapy is to follow and assist the body's great wisdom as it heals and reintegrates after illness. This case illustrates the great power of the protocols to unite the client with his path to wellness.

Doris Weiner, RMT
Plano, Texas
CranioSacral Therapy Practitioner since 2000

A Feather on the Breath of God

❀ I have been doing CranioSacral Therapy for less than a year, but in that time I have probably done at least one hundred applications on my clients and family. Some of the results have been remarkable.

CranioSacral Therapy (CST) relieved my nephew's migraines. He was amazed and told everyone about it. One of my first clients, a friend and fellow massage therapist, had a SomatoEmotional Release. It was quite astounding, since I had no previous experience with it. I did, however, know her past, and she knew that she was in a safe place. I was very open and ready and took the time needed for her to release.

One CranioSacral Therapy client, who is a Reiki therapist and very spiritually in touch, gave this testimony:

"I am a sixty-eight-year-old woman who has been under the care of a chiropractor for the past thirty-five years. My major complaint has always been my neck. I would experience some relief, but the adjustments never lasted for any amount of time.

"I was introduced to CranioSacral Therapy a few months ago. At that time I had strained my neck at the gym. I had been going weekly for adjustments without any real relief. After the first CST session I felt immediate relief and was without any discomfort for a month. I have had two additional sessions and feel that Cranio-Sacral Therapy is definitely for me. Along with alleviating pain, it gives me a general feeling of well-being."

I believe that we have a most wonderful body created by God, and CranioSacral Therapy is a most wonderful helper to keep the body in balance. I am in awe of the profound effects CranioSacral Therapy has on the body and the mind. I receive as much of a blessing from it as my clients do, because it puts me in a very relaxed and meditative state. I hope to learn more about it and how to read the body even better, for CST is a wonderful healing tool.

Susan Hetrick, NCTMB
Waretown, New Jersey
CranioSacral Therapy Practitioner since 2003

Portal to the Superconscious

✿ Joyce came to see me for chronic headaches that she had been having for years. On the phone she told me that she knew there was a "deeper" cause of her headaches and was ready to know what that was.

The day she came to see me, Joyce had a headache, as usual. As she tried to relax on my treatment table, the room suddenly seemed close and still. The look on her face told me that she was excited and hopeful. I carefully explained that I didn't know exactly what would take place during her session, but I did have very strong intentions for her healing. She agreed to just be open and receive whatever healing and guidance came through for her.

I placed my hands under her head and began releasing her cranial base. No sooner did I feel the first release of the muscle tissue at the back of her neck than she went deeply into still point. The hair on the back of my neck rose as I was guided to her abdomen.

I asked Joyce if she had been having any stomach problems, or anything related to her cycle. Tears began to softly run down her cheeks. Soon she was sobbing, and through her tears she told me of her hysterectomy seven years earlier. She felt as if the doctors had betrayed her, that she hadn't really needed the surgery, and it had been done for the sake of convenience. She had regretted it ever since. I asked her if she had ever grieved for her lost body parts and womanhood. She answered that she had cried a lot but hadn't gotten any further than that.

Joyce immediately got very quiet, and I shifted my hands to the position I was guided to. She took a very deep breath, and her cranial rhythm stopped—still point. Then she took another deep breath, and her eyelids fluttered and opened. In this moment her face was soft and angelic. I asked her how she was feeling. "No more headache!" she exclaimed.

I received an e-mail of gratitude from Joyce two months later.

She let me know that a few days after our session, she had taken some time for a grieving ritual that left her feeling free of the anger and resentment from her surgery. And guess what—no headaches in over two months!

Amber Wolf, PhD
Longmont, Colorado
CranioSacral Therapy Practitioner since 1996

New York City Trauma Relief Program

❀ I feel my friend's strong shoulder next to mine, her warmth, her sorrow. It is a cold December evening, and though the rest of the city is decorating for Christmas, there is little cause for joy here. We are walking down Greenwich Street, heading toward an eerie space filled with artificial light and smoke. This is Ground Zero.

Mary and I are here for the week to volunteer our time to the CranioSacral Therapy trauma relief project. On Monday morning we would join a team of CranioSacral Therapists to work with those tender, traumatized survivors who had experienced firsthand the attack on September 11. Not on TV, like Mary and I, but with their own eyes, ears, and bodies. We all would be forced to imagine it all too vividly that whole week, as we listened to and embraced every detail from those who were there.

Christine, a young woman working on the seventy-third floor of the south tower, is making her way down the steps when the second plane hits. She curls on the floor in a corner, certain she will die. A little later, having escaped the building, she hears it begin to fall and thinks it is another bomb. Terrified, she hides in the closet of a nearby friend's apartment.

Fern is running from the collapsing building, but she has muscular dystrophy and cannot run fast enough. She is sure she will be killed. Audrey, stepping out of a subway exit, looks up and sees the first plane slamming into the side of the north tower in front of her. Then comes the second plane. She sees things falling from the upper floors. Horror follows as she realizes they are the flailing arms and legs of human beings as they plummet to their certain deaths. The black ocean of tumbling smoke chases her down the street as she runs for her life. It stops before it reaches her, tumbling in on itself like a wave of water. She is surprised to find herself alive.

Ann is in her bathroom brushing her teeth, her back turned to the view of the WTC towers from her window. She hears the scream of a jet's engine fly close overhead and thinks to herself, "That's too low." She turns and sees the first plane hit the building that has been her view forever. She watches in horror as the whole attack plays out in front of her eyes.

Bob, working in the building next to the WTC towers, hears the first plane hit. Wondering what he heard, he runs out onto the street to see the second plane hit the other tower, the one in which his daughter-in-law Julie works. In terror he realizes that she has probably been killed. She is blind—how could she possibly get out? Then he hears the command to run; the building is falling. For five hours he believes Julie is dead. Finally, he reaches his wife, who tells him that Julie made it out and will meet him uptown. When he sees her alive, he collapses into her arms sobbing. Julie never knew until then how much her husband's family loved her.

Susan, the mother of a two-year-old son, lies on my treatment table and calmly tells me, her beautiful chin quivering, that her husband was one of the firemen killed that day. When she first heard of the attack, she was grateful that Tom was stationed on Staten Island and would be safe. Then came the moment she saw the firehouse chaplain approaching her front door, and she knew. Later she would go to Ground Zero. She found some comfort in seeing that his death was probably instantaneous, that he most likely did not suffer. She shared with me her anger at his choosing to go into the building, choosing work over keeping himself safe for his family. She told me of his brotherhood of fellow firemen and how they had come to help her every day—putting up the Christmas tree, changing the bulb on the porch, filling out insurance papers. She told me of her faith. I did not tell her that her mourning had just begun.

My fellow therapists and I spent day after day listening to the stories, holding the sobbing and those unable to sob. There were policemen, rescuers, teachers from a nearby school, people in the buildings, horrified witnesses, and counselors whose own hearts were breaking. We touched their bodies where they held their horror, their terror, their grief, their disbelief, and their pain. As they softened and let go of their pain, so were we able to let go of ours. We all healed to some measure that week. We all left a little bit lighter, more relaxed, less chaotic and fearful.

It was some of the most difficult, intense, deeply rewarding, and profoundly moving work I have ever done in my life. I feel grateful and privileged to have been invited to participate in the healing of these tender, wounded souls. I am eternally grateful for the gifts of this work.

In a meeting late in the week, one of the therapists likened it to being "called to arms." Our arms—holding, listening, caring, loving. I thank God for that opportunity. I also thank the people who made it possible for me to be there.

Penny Rhodes, CMT, CST-D
Allentown, Pennsylvania
CranioSacral Therapy Practitioner since 1988

9/11: NYC Trauma Intervention

❁ I'm a CranioSacral Therapist practicing in the suburbs of New York. It's December 20, 2001, and I'm on the train heading to NYC to join The Upledger Institute 9/11 trauma intervention team.

I reach the Swedish Institute of Massage Therapy, where thirty Upledger-trained CranioSacral Therapists are working in a large room with about twelve tables. My first client is Joanie.

Joanie lives in Battery Park City, four blocks from Ground Zero. She was at home with her two-year-old son that morning. Hearing the loud crash, she raced to the window. Every person on the street below was standing completely still—all looking in the same direction, all with the same look of horror on their faces. She knew she had to get going. Quickly placing the baby in the stroller, she went out and began to run with everyone else up the West Side Highway—a task made more difficult by the constant shaking she experienced from Parkinson's disease. That day, though, she took certain solace in seeing that everyone was shaking.

My one o'clock appointment hasn't shown up. It's one-thirty, so I begin assisting another therapist whose table is across from the door. I notice a woman and man peering in the window. I go to the door. "She has a one o'clock appointment," he says. "She's late."

"Marcia gave me her appointment," the woman says. "My name is Faith." She keeps looking down at the floor, fixing her gaze at her feet. Leading her to my table at the opposite end of the room, I notice that she never looks up once. I'm joined by another therapist, and we begin to work.

"I'm having panic attacks," Faith says. "They started about a month ago." We discover that she's suffering from agoraphobia (fear of going out), and that's why her boyfriend has accompanied her.

"It's just too much. I'm moving out of the city with my son

Steven. He's three. I can't handle it alone. I can't sleep. I want to give up. The last time this happened was ten years ago. It was too much then, too."

Going back, we uncover issues stemming from when she was three years old. It proves a long trip back from there to the present. When we are through, Faith decides that all she needs are a couple of people to move in with her there in New York. She needs to trust, though.

"Trust takes more work," she says. "Sometimes it's easier to go with fear. It's more familiar, and I get to fall apart. With trust, I have to take the next step. Okay, I can do that."

Once we are finished, she says, "Oh, so that's what this room looks like. I didn't dare look before." She leaves upbeat, looking at the world with interest, light in her face.

One of the therapists tells me about Jessica. Jessica worked on the seventy-second floor of Two World Trade Center. When the first plane hit, she curled up under her desk in the fetal position in terror, thinking she was going to die. Then she ran down seventy-two flights of stairs in three-inch heels. Over the loudspeaker she heard, "Return to your office. You are perfectly safe."

On the street, Jessica ran with everyone else. She ran to her boss's house. They heard planes overhead and thought the attack was continuing. She hid in the closet curled up in the fetal position again.

The therapist says, "We just kept releasing layer after layer of fear. So much fear kept coming out of her."

Fran lives downtown. She has experienced stomach problems since September 11th. She has been to the doctor, but it hasn't helped. We identify fear living in her stomach. We ask how long it has been there, but she doesn't know. I try dating its origins the way Visceral Manipulation developer Jean-Pierre Barral, DO, teaches how to date a scar. I got a fuzzy indication that it was between the ages of seven and fourteen years. Picking an age, I ask her, "What was going on when you were ten?"

She is quiet and then says, "I can't think of anything."

We go on to do structural work at the liver, stomach, and kidneys. She then tells me that she grew up in Jerusalem.

"We began sleeping in a bomb shelter at night," she says. "But none of that was unusual. I'm surprised to find fear around from that time. I didn't think it affected me anymore. Why did I feel so much shock when I saw the towers go down? I thought I'd be used to it by now. I thought I'd be numb."

So she pictures herself sitting down with Fear in our waiting room and talking with it. Fear shrugs and says to her, "What did you expect?" She laughs.

Another therapist tells us about treating Laurie, who is eight weeks pregnant. He says, "Here she is, bringing a new baby into the world, the new generation, and I couldn't find any fear in her body at all. None. I was so happy, filled with hope. She was delivering a baby into the world, and she was completely fearless. I told her that she was the start of a new breed of New Yorkers. Completely fearless."

It is Friday, the end of the day. Tad Wanveer, LMT, CST-D (UI HealthPlex clinician who is heading the program), tells us that we've treated around one hundred people, and the response is overwhelmingly positive.

In particular, most everyone mentions how much it means to them that therapists from as far away as Ireland have come to help. We decide that in any future program, this would be something we would like to continue. It gives us all the feeling that our trauma is shared.

Elizabeth Pasquale, LMT, CST
Ossining, New York
CranioSacral Therapy Practitioner since 1998

Make Peace with God and Fly

❋ One CranioSacral Therapy session that will always stay with me occurred on the last day of the trauma relief program we did in New York after 9/11.

I was working with Chas Perry, PhD, CST-D, and John Rollinson, EdD, CST. Our first patient was Audrey, who had been asked to return for a second session. She was a tall, beautiful young woman who worked in the fashion industry. She was struggling to continue each day because so many areas of her life were crippled by the collapse of the World Trade Center.

We asked Audrey about her first session. She said it had been very profound, but she had cried for most of that day and the next. She was having a hard time processing so much.

I had worked with her lead therapist from her first session, and I knew that this practitioner was incredibly nurturing and comforting. This had helped Audrey get to the place where she could now gain some perspective and understanding of how the events of 9/11 could be integrated into her life.

After we arced, Chas began to work on her upper neck area; John was working with her left hip and sacrum; and I was working first with her lungs and then her heart. As we all settled into the tissue, she began to cry quietly.

She told us that on 9/11 she had come up from the subway just after the first plane hit the building. She was stunned. Then she saw the second plane hit. As both buildings were in flames, she didn't know what to do. She watched in horror as people ran past her and as others began to jump from the buildings to escape the fires. She remembered seeing one man, in particular, pausing on the ledge of a building before he jumped many stories to his certain death.

In that moment, three months later, her feelings had shifted to incredible, deep sadness and grief over the people she had seen jumping from the buildings. They had had no time to reconcile their lives, no time to say good-bye; they had simply reacted.

Audrey had gone back to her apartment and watched the news with some friends, crying and shaking from all the events beyond her door and her neighborhood.

A few days after 9/11, she went to the Colorado River for a rafting trip with some friends. She had some mixed feelings about leaving but was committed to her plans. She told of pausing on the river, looking back at her friends, and feeling a deep connection. She relayed moving metaphors about the river and her life, and how her friends had challenged and supported her. It was a moving journey she took us on as she recounted her days on the river.

Next, she told us about her dearly loved uncle who had died recently after a long illness. He left no unresolved business, no one he had not told "I love you." He had been brave and calm as he faced death, and she clearly admired his courage.

Faced with the contrast of her uncle's quiet passing and the horror of the figures jumping from buildings, Audrey wept. She was able to find some perspective, however, through her uncle's courage. At one point these words came to her: "Make peace with God and fly." She connected with the particular man on the ledge, the one she had seen pausing. She was able to see that perhaps in his moment of hesitation he was making peace with God and his life, and that he flew.

During this session, Audrey's pericardium, the heart protector, was tight and restricted. As she wept and connected to her uncle, there was some freedom in the tissue. Her neck softened while Chas worked with some regional tissue release, and as John and I connected on the posterior and anterior sides of her heart.

She also told us that she had been having difficulty eating and sleeping. Remarkably, each time she connected more closely to her heart and it softened, there was a reciprocal rumbling in her stomach. Clearly, the two were intimately related. Chas ended the session quietly with some visceral work for her stomach.

Audrey's experience was intense and deep, as was her session that day. We exceeded our two hours, and I was struck by the connection between we three therapists and this woman. All of us played a critical role in supporting Audrey as she unraveled the rich layers of emotion she had experienced.

At the end of our sessions on the final day in New York, the therapists gathered in a circle before parting. We went around and shared our thoughts about the week. Audrey's words stayed with me, and I felt they could lend some perspective for all of us. I said, from this point on, what is left is to make peace with God about the events of 9/11, along with the events in our lives, and then go on to the next place. It is now time to fly.

Sally Morgan, PT, CST, TTEAM
Northampton, Massachusetts
CranioSacral Therapy Practitioner since 1994

Everything Is Connected

In 1998 I had a patient named Susan come to see me. She could barely walk a straight line due to a car accident. Her left temporal bone had hit numerous times on the driver's-side window, resulting in a right lateral strain. She complained about cluster headaches along with eye-motor and visual dysfunctions. She had a hard time focusing her eyes. She indicated that she had difficulty remembering what she had done minutes before. Her husband complained about a personality dysfunction.

When I palpated both temporals, the left one was concave and right one convex. I started to work on the sphenoid using Cranio-Sacral Therapy (CST). As soon as the sphenoid was corrected, Susan could read the four-inch print on a poster that I had hanging on the wall. She hadn't been able to read it prior.

Next I worked on the temporals and mandible with all the techniques I had learned. Susan was hearing and seeing better. Her mandible was straight bilaterally, and chewing was now on each side of her mouth.

She kept complaining about a severe pain that was going from the left to the right ASIS, to the midline, up the sternum, and to the left aspect of the face, where there was tremendous pain. Where did this pain come from?

While working on the lower leg one day, I felt it start to internally rotate. All of a sudden, Susan started remembering the accident like a quick dream. She said, "My foot is caught under the car seat where I'm sitting. The pain is so great!" She then proceeded to tell me in medical terms where, exactly, the pain was going. I had never heard her speak this way, but the information was certainly helpful.

I stayed with the lower leg for half an hour. Next I put my two fingers lightly on the sphenoid, which sent Susan into orbit. The pain had now taken the reverse route right down to her ankle, which was now internally rotated. She placed my fingers on her sphenoid again and stayed with the feeling. She discovered the connection at the root of her headache. In two treatments the pain route was gone. Susan walked without the constant pain in her body and face.

Joan L. Mailing, RMT
Brantford, Ontario, Canada
CranioSacral Therapy Practitioner since 1997

Your Health Is Your Wealth

❀ The birth of my youngest son eight years ago left me with a chronically sore back. Chiropractic, exercise, and massage therapy did little to relieve the tension and pain. It felt as if a wire were holding my back and the sacral area stiff.

After receiving CranioSacral Therapy (CST), my back pain dissipated and my spine and neck experienced greatly decreased tension. CST went so much deeper than the other approaches, and there were no painful after-effects—just a little stiffness that went away in two days.

The CranioSacral Therapy coursework I have taken has given me personal growth beyond any level I could understand. During a particular session, I processed the trauma from being struck by lightning when I was two years old. That was forty years ago!

I had run out of the house during the beginning of a rainstorm. My mom and sister were frantically taking laundry off the clothesline. I was by a light pole in our yard when the lightning struck. My breathing stopped. My mom picked me up and shook me while she was crying, calling my name, "Wendy, are you okay?" I gasped and cried in mom's arms.

After this CranioSacral Therapy session, I had increased energy and felt a heavy weight come off my chest.

Overall, CranioSacral Therapy has made daily activities of living much easier. My thinking is clearer and more focused. And I have increased mobility in my spine and musculoskeletal system.

Every day I look forward to introducing at least one new client to the experience of CranioSacral Therapy. I truly feel my health has been enhanced, and I passionately pass this on to clients.

One of these clients was a thirty-seven-year-old female massage therapist who had experienced progressively worsening back pain for at least ten years. The sacrum would rotate left and cause much pain in the lumbar area.

Once a month for a year this client had been treated with the usual massage techniques that worked the musculature of the low back, gluteal, psoas, etc. Within three weeks after each treatment, though, the back would reposition to the painful status.

I explained CranioSacral Therapy to her, applied the techniques, and we have not looked back since. This client's back problem has resolved, and she keeps regular monthly CST appointments.

This client loves it when I come back from another course. I always have new methods to help her experience further blending and melding, which provides her system a holistic approach to self-regeneration and alignment.

The world today needs an increased preventative measure to ensure ultimate health—for health is wealth! CranioSacral Therapy on a regular basis promotes a well-tuned, functioning nervous system, which leads to decreased stress, increased immunity, and, ultimately, a healthy mind and body. What more could we want?!

Wendy Gambrel, MT
Winnipeg, Manitoba, Canada
CranioSacral Therapy Practitioner since 2002

Good Intention, Strong Will:
A Winning Combination

Michael was twenty-eight years old when I first saw him try to handle the cash register at my local health food store. The poor guy wore glasses as thick as old Coke bottles, yet still had to hold the price stickers up to his nose to read the numbers. I spoke to him about the possible benefits of CranioSacral Therapy, although it was uncertain whether it would work with his condition.

Michael had been diagnosed with nystagmus and had never been able to hold a job, live anywhere other than his parents' house, or drive himself places. Of secondary concern was intermittent pain in various areas of his body.

His dependence on everyone around him, although necessary, bothered Michael. He was willing to try CranioSacral Therapy and committed to ten sessions. These were conducted for the most part on a weekly basis.

Michael was fascinating to work on. The physical changes included pain reduction; vision improvement, though slight and probably due to the reduction in the rapid and constant movement of his eyes; elimination of the red, swollen eyes that gave the initial impression of drug abuse; improved balance so that he was now confident enough to walk across a field without stumbling; and resumption of upper- and lower-body integration at vertebrae level L5/S1 [lumbar vertebra, sacral vertebra].

While all of this was wonderful and fulfilling for me as a therapist, the story his girlfriend told me a short time after treatment stopped will never leave me. Dear Michael found a sense of confidence he had never felt before. He bought a truck, drove himself (with his girlfriend driving behind him in her vehicle) all the way to Colorado, signed his first lease for an apartment, and secured a job as a carpenter's apprentice. Wow!

Nancy S.C. Thomer, CMT
Pipersville, Pennsylvania
CranioSacral Therapy Practitioner since 1991

A New Outlook for Bert

✿ Bert was an eighty-three-year-old resident of a skilled nursing facility at the time of this story. Available medical/surgical information on him was scanty. What was known was that he had multiple medical conditions too numerous to mention. Among them were arthritis, depression, and documented chronic neck pain. The doctors had told Bert that the only way to correct his pain was with surgery, but that he was not a surgical candidate because of his health problems and advanced age.

The nursing staff reported that Bert was often cranky—downright cantankerous at times—and spent most of the day in his room alone. He was not able to move his head into an upright position; it was flexed downward so that he was looking at his lap.

During his daily morning walks, assisted by a staff person and using a walker, he could not see where he was going and simply watched his feet move one in front of the other. When his daughter took him for a ride in the car, he stared at his lap and could not see over the dashboard. No wonder he was out of sorts! What a depressing and lonely way to exist.

After a new therapy company began providing services at the facility, Bert asked to be seen by a therapist on the chance that something could be done to ease his pain. The financial burden of therapy was covered only partially by insurance, but he was willing to do anything to try and get some relief. Some of the nursing staff warned me that he might be difficult or grouchy, but they were also pleased that I was willing to give it a try.

I saw Bert a total of fourteen sessions over the course of four weeks. When we began treatment, he needed moderate to maximum assistance from two people to help him assume a supine position on the air mattress, which had been placed on the treatment table. We needed to prop up his head with three pillows so that he was semi-comfortable and breathing was not challenged too much.

(In his own bed he slept on his side with his head curled into his chest.)

At our initial evaluation, Bert reported pain in his neck and lumbar spine. He showed generalized stiffness and lack of mobility in all major joints. He had flexion of thirty degrees at rest; no neck extension; little to no rotation or lateral flexion to either side of his neck; and was capable of being passively ranged to fifteen degrees from neutral. Bert's craniosacral rhythm was weak, indicating little excursion, vitality, or volume; it was almost impalpable in the lower extremities.

Treatment sessions loosely followed the CranioSacral Therapy 10-Step Protocol. Applications consisted of diaphragm releases, with each diaphragm being the focus of one or more sessions; regional/positional tissue releases of all four extremities and neck; movement of the cranial bones, especially the sphenoid, temporals, and occiput; SomatoEmotional Releases, which included some tears and sad memories that were not described verbally in any length; and direction of energy, especially at the neck and lower spine.

By the end of treatment, a number of changes had taken place. Bert's neck position at rest was between neutral and ten degrees extension. He now needed only one pillow to be comfortable lying down. He was able to rotate his neck fifteen degrees to the left and twenty degrees to the right. He jokingly reported that he could now turn his head to flirt with women in the hallway. Bert said he had no pain in his low back or neck. He demonstrated more freedom of movement (less joint stiffness), as evidenced by his ability to transfer himself from his wheelchair to and from the mat table with moderate assistance. His craniosacral rhythm was stronger, with greater excursion, and indicated palpably increased strength and vitality.

The nursing staff observed changes in Bert's mobility when he was seated in his wheelchair, improved balance and speed during ambulation, and a noticeable improvement in his overall mood.

To say that treatment was successful would not begin to describe the benefits of using a CranioSacral Therapy approach with Bert. He so looked forward to each day he was to have therapy that he would wait outside the room for an hour before his scheduled appointment.

I could spend hours describing each session's changes and the profound words of appreciation expressed by Bert each and every time I worked with him. No matter what I say, though, the results can best be summarized by Bert himself. The following was dictated by him several days after his last session.

"Therapy went way above all my expectations. There was no pain; it was just so gentle and kind. The pain in my neck was terrible, and the doctors told me the only way to fix it was with surgery, but I couldn't have any. Mary Helen fixed my neck and the pain is gone. She got my head 'screwed on straight,' so now I can see where I am going, and I'm not looking down at the floor. This was the most wonderful experience of my life! Thank you for making me feel better. You have given me back my life."

Mary Helen Young, MS, OTR/L
Grovesport, Ohio
CranioSacral Therapy Practitioner since 1994

Fighting Breast Cancer with CST

My story begins in 1993 when I was the supervisor of eighteen therapists at a private pediatric clinic.

I was putting in long days *and* long nights, as my mother had come to live with us. I wasn't taking care of myself, so when I got the shingles I wasn't surprised, just annoyed. When I repeatedly got cysts in my left breast, I had them needled and kept going.

Then a lump appeared that couldn't be needled. The surgeon recommended a lumpectomy biopsy to determine what type of cells the lump contained. The surgery was a relatively simple procedure, and my surgeon told me that I had abnormal cells but no cancer. That was a relief, because my mom had gone through breast cancer the year before. I felt I had dodged a bullet.

My health issues did not end after the lumpectomy. I started going through menopause, complete with night sweats, hot flashes, and anxiety attacks. I needed relief but didn't find it by going to traditional doctors. They wouldn't put me on hormone-replacement therapy because of the abnormal cells in my breast. I began reading about nutrition and menopause and started to get some relief through dietary changes.

In 1996 a flyer on CranioSacral Therapy came across my desk at work. A therapist friend thought I would like it because it treated the whole person. With my background in Sensory Integration and neurodevelopmental therapy, I have always found that whole-person approaches hold the most interest for me. I signed up for a class.

CranioSacral Therapy hooked me on the second day of class when a blocked sinus I had been dealing with for months cleared up when the instructor did a frontal lift on me. I couldn't wait to take more classes.

As the many blocks in my body cleared, my health improved. I left my job in corporate therapy and started working for myself.

Every course got me more excited about the work, and each new patient became a wonderful teacher. This spurred me on to get better and better at holding space for their bodies to heal. To sit in awe of the body's ability to heal has been my best job ever.

In 2002 I had the privilege of working with Dr. Lisa Upledger as part of the advanced clinical applications program at The Upledger Institute. In the afternoon we each received multiple-therapist hands-on treatments.

I had found a lump in my left breast just before I left for Florida and was scheduled for a biopsy when I got back home. A number of emotional issues came to the surface at this time. Through these sessions I made peace with my breasts.

I wasn't prepared for my biopsy results. The scar tissue from my 1993 biopsy contained invasive cancer. I went for a second opinion at the Dana Farber Cancer Center in Boston. They confirmed the diagnosis and said that the original slides had been read incorrectly. I had ductal carcinoma *in situ,* but the surgeons hadn't gotten clean margins when they did the lumpectomy.

My first thought was "I've had cancer for nine years!" My second thought was "Thank God for all the changes I've made in my life since 1993. I've got a fighting chance to beat this disease."

I had a dream the month before the biopsy. In the dream I had scars on both sides of my chest, but I was alive and happy. Trusting the dream as Divine Intervention, I told my surgeon that I wanted both breasts removed. Since my mother also experienced breast cancer, he said he would remove and biopsy both breasts. I also told him that I wanted my friend, Pam McCormack, a CranioSacral Therapist, to treat me in pre-op so that I would go into surgery relaxed and without Valium. He agreed to this request and the surgery went well.

When I got back to my room Pam and two other friends were there to continue the CranioSacral Therapy. When my doctor came to see me at six p.m. he said I didn't look like a patient. I told him that I was only taking Tylenol for the pain. He was surprised and mentioned that there would be a prescription for stronger medication at the nurses' station. I never needed it. I was ready to go home the next morning with four drains in place. I healed quickly and never needed anything stronger than Tylenol.

The biopsy results from the surgery showed that I had invasive cancer in both breasts but only one positive lymph node. The oncologist recommended four rounds of chemotherapy. I agreed to do this because my breast had felt like a hornets' nest after the biopsy, and I wanted to make sure all the cancer cells were eliminated.

I told Pam that her services would be needed again. I had her treat me the next day to help me deal with the effects of chemo. She saw me at my worst. I couldn't believe how horrible the chemo made me feel and how good it felt to be treated.

Each session of chemo was worse than the one before. After the third session my white blood count dropped dangerously low and stayed down. I decided that my body was telling me not to do a fourth treatment. After I told my oncologist, my blood count jumped drastically. I again felt Divinely guided.

Two years after this experience I feel great and have a very busy therapy practice. I still get occasional treatments and continue to have releases around the whole experience. I am happily assisting others through the cancer experience with CranioSacral Therapy and Lymph Drainage Therapy. Life is good!

Lorna Kerbel, PT, CST, LLCC
Wilbraham, Massachusetts
CranioSacral Therapy Practitioner since 1996

Hysterectomy Avoided with CST

❀ As a massage therapist, I have recommended CranioSacral Therapy (CST) to others. It is my personal experience with the therapy, however, that is most remarkable.

I was diagnosed with a ten-centimeter ovarian cyst. My doctor performed laparoscopy and discovered that my entire pelvic region was full of adhesions. Along with the cyst, he also removed a tube and ovary. During my next pap smear, irregular cells were found, and loop excision was performed. The cells were found to be benign. As a result of all the reproductive problems, I was told that I had chronic pelvic inflammatory disease.

I generally experienced severe pelvic pain and bloating three weeks out of every month. The doctor's only suggestion was for me to have a hysterectomy or again undergo laparoscopy to remove the other tube and any new adhesions. This only gave a fifty–fifty chance for improvement.

Terribly desperate, I almost agreed to surgery. When Jasuti Goss showed me literature indicating that CranioSacral Therapy could help alleviate pelvic pain, I remained skeptical. I decided that I had nothing to lose, so I would try the treatment with Jasuti.

The day following the session, I felt euphoric and energized. My next menstrual cycle produced only three days of normal discomfort, and I no longer had to consider having a hysterectomy.

More than one year later, I still experience only normal discomfort during menstrual cycles.

Story by Lisa Oakes, CMT
Submitted by Jasuti Goss, NCMT
Anderson, Indiana
CranioSacral Therapy Practitioner since 1998

Planting the Seeds of CST

❀ In 1990 I suffered for eleven months with chronic fatigue. Then in 1995 it reared its ugly head again after my first miscarriage. Several times my mother made mention of a new therapy from an institute in South Florida that would help with my chronic fatigue. I listened politely then ignored her advice.

Continuing to feel awful, I finally went for a CranioSacral Therapy (CST) treatment in Orlando, where someone from the institute was visiting. I had perhaps two or three CST sessions along with massage therapy.

Soon I was pregnant again, delivering full term in 1996 with a C-section. While I was pregnant with this baby, my mother gave me a book from The Upledger Institute about CranioSacral Therapy. After reading it, I had a much better appreciation for how life-changing it can be; but being busy with a newborn, I stored away the information.

Over the next five years the chronic fatigue wasn't taking center stage in my life, but having another successful pregnancy was. After three difficult miscarriages (one in the first trimester and the other two in the early second trimester), seeing an infertility specialist and chiropractor, and taking the infertility drug Clomid, my husband and I decided to stop trying to have a second child. After the last miscarriage, one of the comments I remember hearing from the doctor was that the fetus was not getting adequate blood supply.

I went back on the pill and my husband was about to schedule a vasectomy when I got pregnant! We were scared to death. I was being treated for an auto accident at the time with chiropractic and massage therapy. I told my massage therapist that I was pregnant again and let it be known that this baby was going to go full term. I was within weeks of being forty and had had four miscarriages. What were the chances of a successful full-term pregnancy?

I did my part, eating healthy, keeping my stress level down, getting proper rest, etc. I believe, however, that my daughter would not be here today if she had not had my therapist's gifted hands. She treated my unborn daughter and me with CranioSacral Therapy from the beginning of my pregnancy until my daughter was delivered in the hospital.

As my therapist worked on the two of us, I meditated on having a successful delivery. The baby was always very responsive during our sessions, rolling and tumbling in the womb. When I left my CranioSacral sessions I always felt calm, relaxed, and peaceful. When my therapist treated my newborn with CST in the hospital, I know she knew her touch. How blessed is that little girl!

The baby thrived throughout the pregnancy, and there is no doubt in my mind that she thrived and developed due to CranioSacral Therapy. I also have to thank my therapist for my daughter's activity level. She always smiles, is happy, and never stops talking, walking, running, or jumping. She was so spoiled in the womb! CST definitely got the blood flowing to her. If only the doctor knew the real reason why she is here today. I do believe that God, my therapist, and I made this happen ... well, my hubby might have had something to do with it, too!

Submitted by Barbara Nelen, LMT
Winter Park, Florida
CranioSacral Therapy Practitioner since 1997

The Sledding Accident

❁ The CranioSacral Therapy (CST) workshop I took in January 1999 still holds a strong memory for me. Though I had been doing this work since 1996, I decided to take a refresher course.

The class was filled with interesting people in the healthcare field. In addition to the lecture, we had some hands-on training. The instructor explained how people can relive incidents.

It was time to begin working on each other. The instructor asked us to pick a partner for exchanging treatments. Another massage therapist and I, seated next to each other, chose to work together for the hands-on practice. She worked on me first. I had some small releases. I explained to her that I had been getting CST since 1995.

After she finished it was my turn to do the 10-Step Protocol on her. We both felt some releases in her head as I placed my hands in various specified positions. Her body was responding well to the treatment.

Neither one of us was prepared for the next release. Her brain was constricted, and we both felt a big release. With this major release she became emotionally upset, and she began to shake violently as if going into shock. Her temperature began to drop, and she said she was freezing cold. Her body looked like it was freezing, as if she were really outside in very cold weather.

I immediately put a blanket around her, and another student brought a second blanket. Seeing the commotion, the instructor came over. I kept talking to my practice partner during this time in a calming voice, letting her know that she was safe and I was present for her. Within a very short period of time her body relaxed.

After a few minutes she explained her experience. She told us that as she felt the constriction release, she had a vivid memory of a sledding accident with her brother when she was a little girl. She had been told by her mother not to go sledding but had decided to go anyway. During one run, her brother lost control of the sled and they hit a big tree. She was hurt, bleeding, very cold, and was shaking. All the while she was in great emotional turmoil because her mother had told her not to go, and she was afraid of Mother's reaction to her disobedience.

Besides being a massage therapist, I have a background in crisis intervention. I definitely used those tools that day. None of my CST treatments before or after has been so intense. The great news about this incident was that we felt a human bond. We had gone through something together. We both experienced her physical reaction held from her childhood. Her body and mind remembered and relived the incident. My hands felt the cold body; my eyes saw her anguish.

The experience changed both our lives. It gave me a deeper respect for the body. It left both of us with a deep feeling of a shared experience and a level of trust.

Anne Marie McNamara, LMT
Seattle, Washington
CranioSacral Therapy Practitioner since 1996

Wake Up and Smell the Coffee!

I began working with Ms. C in January of 2003 for pain she was experiencing in her neck, back, and arms. She had been diagnosed with carpal tunnel syndrome, most likely associated with her twenty-four years as a dental hygienist. Other symptoms included longstanding psoriasis and high levels of stress.

I treated Ms. C with deep tissue massage, neuromuscular therapy, myofascial therapy, stretching, and postural exercises. These techniques were helpful in reducing her symptoms but also left her extremely sore for more than a week following the session. She was very receptive to alternate methods of treatment, so I suggested CranioSacral Therapy (CST), both as a method of relieving her pain with less tissue trauma and as a possible way to address her psoriasis symptoms and overall stress.

At this point, I must mention that I had completed my first CranioSacral Therapy class on April 6, 2003. On April 11, Ms. C and I experienced her first CST session, which consisted of CV-4 and diaphragm-release techniques. I attempted to release her frontal bone, but I felt unable to obtain a full release.

One week later, at her next session, Ms. C mentioned an improvement in her sense of smell, to which I replied, "That's nice—was there anything wrong with it to begin with?" To my astonishment, she told me the following story.

When she was pregnant with her daughter twenty-four years prior, Ms. C had passed out and hit her head on the corner of a table, sustaining a closed-head injury. Since that time, she had been unable to smell. Her doctor told her that her nerve was permanently damaged and she would be unable to smell again.

Subsequent CST sessions restored her sense of smell entirely. She was elated that she could actually smell her coffee in the morning!

This incident happened over a year ago, and I can recall it as clearly as if it were yesterday. To me it illustrates the awesome healing power of CranioSacral Therapy. If a novice practitioner, five days out of her first course, can use these techniques and release the body's amazing capacity to heal itself, imagine what practitioners with more experience and knowledge can accomplish!

Ms. C's experience inspired me to continue my CranioSacral Therapy training. I am applying to become a teaching assistant and have begun the process to become Techniques-certified.

Thank you, Ms. C, for inspiring me to continue my own process of growth. Thank you, Dr. Upledger, for the unique opportunities you have given us to assist the body in utilizing its wonderful healing potential.

Alice G. Huss, PT, LMT, CPI
Albuquerque, New Mexico
CranioSacral Therapy Practitioner since 2003

The Connection

✿ Over the last nine years, I've watched the man who taught me some of life's greatest lessons fight cancer with the greatest tenacity. Although my stepfather in name, he is Dad in my heart. His name is Frank Champa, and he taught me what it means to love and be loved unconditionally; what it means to sacrifice and give of yourself; what it means to help someone no matter how small it may seem at the time; and what it means to have faith.

Nine years ago, my dad was diagnosed with prostate cancer. By the time it was discovered, it had spread throughout his lymph system. Three years ago he also developed a massive brain tumor that was completely unrelated to the prostate cancer. In less than a decade, he underwent chemotherapy, radiation, numerous test-trial medications, hormone therapy, brain surgery, anti-seizure medications, steroids, sedatives, anti-nausea medication, and mind-altering pain medicines too powerful to speak of.

As a CranioSacral Therapy provider, I had great difficulty trying to emotionally separate myself and be in the state I needed to be in to treat Dad. Instead, I asked a friend to treat him, and I also took him to the UI HealthPlex clinic during a visit to Florida.

Several months ago, there was another setback. His medications had taken a toll on his bowels, rendering him unable to get out of bed because of the pain. There are no words to describe the feeling of helplessness in watching a parent in agony. Without even thinking, I gently laid my hands on his abdomen that day. Blending. Softening. Relaxing. Releasing emotions. Finally he was able to drift off into a peaceful sleep. When he awoke, his pain was greatly lessened, and he was able to get out of bed. He spoke of "healing hands."

My family and I have since lost from this Earth the greatest man we've ever known. I am unable to put into words the ugliness and devastation of brain cancer and the effects it has on loved ones.

One month of sleep deprivation while caring for him and the deep emotions involved left me in a state unsuitable to treat him. I could only be there as his daughter, by his side until the very end.

Although the CranioSacral Therapy I provided Dad a couple of months prior was but a brief pause in the suffering he endured, I was proud to have helped him, and I am grateful that I was able to have that connection.

Shannon Desilets, PT
Pembroke, New Hampshire
CranioSacral Therapy Practitioner since 2002

Life's a Beach

❀ Donna came to me as a "last resort." She had tried just about everything, from no-carb diets to exercise and everything in between, and her symptoms continued to persist. Diagnosed with multiple sclerosis in 1990, her main difficulties were loss of bladder control, situational vertigo, optical neuritis, and weakness in the left leg.

In 1996, after rupturing a disc, Donna underwent three separate back surgeries. Doctors finally put in titanium cages and a screw. They told her that the bone in that area was crumbling like chalk. She experienced recurring inflammation of the spinal nerve in that area and pain into the left leg. Ongoing surgery-related problems with clotting in her legs and lungs necessitated the placement of a Greenfield filter in the vena cava.

Donna was given a diagnosis of fibromyalgia after experiencing episodes of pain dating back to when she was a teenager. The pain became so great that even wearing clothes was painful. She couldn't wear jewelry, and her feet hurt so badly that she bought bigger shoes so her feet wouldn't touch the sides.

When Donna came to my office, her cholesterol was in the range of four hundred to five hundred sixty, with triglycerides at seven hundred ten up to eighteen hundred. Medicine, food, and exercise had resulted in varying degrees of success at different times. While taking Lipitor, her liver enzymes had gone off the charts, and her doctor called her at home to tell her to stop the medication immediately.

Donna tried acupuncture, massage, therapeutic touch, relaxation tapes, exercise (with a personal trainer), weight training, walking, hot baths, ice packs, and medicine. Seeing a psychotherapist on a regular basis helped with the emotional and mental aspects of her diseases.

According to Donna, one of the biggest disappointments was

that for the last seven years, she had not been able to walk on the beach when she visited her mom in Florida. Because the beach slants toward the ocean, walking on the angle caused her great pain.

Donna came to me through a friend who encouraged her to get CranioSacral Therapy (CST). December 1, 2003, was her first treatment, and her response was immediate and profound. "It's the first time in fifty-six years that I feel connected" was her statement.

Donna continued to come in for CST on a regular basis. During many of the sessions she had several SomatoEmotional Releases that got her in touch with traumatic events in her childhood. She says these releases changed her life. She is now more able to see possibilities, knowing there isn't anything in life she can't get through.

By Donna's appointment in March 2004, her cholesterol had dropped dramatically. When her doctor called her with the results, he told her to continue taking whatever medication she was on. Donna's reply was "I'm not taking anything. I'm just getting Cranio-Sacral Therapy." (At this writing Donna's cholesterol has gone up but remains lower than her counts in December 2003.)

Commenting on other positive effects that CranioSacral Therapy has had on her life, Donna claims she is more open, more sensitive, more interested in listening and sharing, and more vulnerable. Her energy level is up, and she has learned how to deal with the pain that comes periodically. She is able to walk for an hour and is running at times. She even plays racquetball, which she hadn't done since 1996.

While Donna enjoys the connection of mind, body, and spirit more than ever before, the real joy came recently on her last visit to her mom's. You guessed it—she walked on the beach for the first time in seven years.

Nancy Costello, LMT
Newport, Kentucky
CranioSacral Therapy Practitioner since 2000

CranioSacral to the Rescue

❁ Walter is a fifty-nine-year-old financial advisor who suffered his first bout of trigeminal neuralgia in April of 2001. According to the *Merck Manual*, "Trigeminal neuralgia is pain due to malfunction of cranial nerve V, which carries sensory information from the face to the brain and controls the muscles involved in chewing."

At first Walter's doctor diagnosed him with sinusitis and said he needed surgery to drain the sinus over his right eye. He went for a second opinion at Massachusetts Eye and Ear and was told that they couldn't determine the cause of his pain, but he didn't need surgery on his sinuses. His doctor then gave him a prescription for Neurontin and referred him to a neurologist.

Two months later Walter was seen by the neurologist. Since the Neurontin had provided no relief, he was switched to Tegretol. This caused his white blood cell count to drop so low that the drug had to be discontinued. The next drug they tried was Trileptal. After his neurologist left the area, a new one added Baclofen.

Walter was still experiencing pain on these drugs, so a consultation with a neurosurgeon was recommended. He suggested that Walter read about the Gamma Knife technique, which uses focused radiation to destroy the nerve and relieve the pain permanently.

A friend of Walter's recommended that he look into nutritional supplements and cranial osteopathy instead of surgery. He located The Upledger Institute's website, where he found my name and gave me a call. He wanted to know if I had worked on anyone with trigeminal neuralgia and if I'd had success treating the condition. He also wanted to know how many treatments he would need. I told him I'd had success with a woman who experienced trigeminal neuralgia after a car accident, but that I couldn't promise he would get the same results. I told him to try six treatments to start, since he had already had the pain for over two years.

Our first session was memorable. Walter arrived looking drawn from lack of sleep and taut from constant pain. As he filled out the questionnaire the smoke detector went off, adding to his discomfort. Once he settled down on the treatment table he could not shut down his left brain. Why did I have my hands on his sacrum? What was I feeling in his body? What did he need to do when the session was over?

Despite all the questions, Walter's body began to release. His cranial rhythm was shallow, asymmetrical, and had very little flexion. His entire right side felt compressed, especially the sacrum and cranial base. We focused on these areas, and he was able to reconnect with himself as an eighteen-year-old, to the time when he was knocked down and hit his head on a sidewalk. This was only one of many stories that Walter's bones, fascia, and organs had to tell.

Walter was pleasantly surprised to learn that his body could speak about the injuries, both physical and emotional, that had occurred throughout his life. The first session ended on a positive note, with decreased pain, so he scheduled more visits.

Walter was treated twice a week, usually by me and colleague Pam McCormack, also a certified CranioSacral Therapist. As his pain continued to decrease in intensity and frequency, we began to see another side of him. He had a good sense of humor and took delight in kidding around with us. This change was primarily due to the fact that, as his pain decreased and his sleep increased, his true nature began to emerge. He often said that he felt we had given him his life back. I reminded Walter that we had simply opened space for his body to do great work.

After four months of treatment Walter began making plans to go abroad. Unfortunately his plans came to a halt when his car was hit by another car. This caused a recurrence of the trigeminal neuralgia, along with typical whiplash symptoms in his back and neck. After another three months of therapy his pain was diminished significantly.

Walter had been instructed in the use of a Still Point Inducer and an herbal wrap for his back. He had established a daily morning routine of stretching and strengthening exercises. He was now ready for his trip.

When Walter returns from his two months abroad he will prob-ably resume therapy at least once a month. There are more stories for his body to tell, and he is an individual ready and willing to do the work.

Lorna Kerbel, PT, CST, LLCC
Wilbraham, Massachusetts
CranioSacral Therapy Practitioner since 1996

Don't Just Control Pain—End It!

❀ My problems started four years ago when I sprained the sacroiliac joint ligaments in my hip/lower back area while doing water aerobics. I went to my doctor, who diagnosed the problem and sent me to a physical therapist. After six weeks of therapy, the pain was still there but under control.

I continued to have flare-ups, which often left me in severe pain and unable to stand up straight. Once again I returned to the doctor. This time he prescribed both muscle relaxant and anti-inflammatory medications. He also put me on bed rest for three to five days and told me to use alternating heat and cold therapy. After following his instructions, I found that the pain returned to a tolerable level, sort of like a nagging toothache. At least I was able to function once again. I learned to live with the pain.

Then in May 2001, the pain started to intensify again, but this time it was different. Not only did I have pain from the sacroiliac joint, but I also had a pinched peroneal nerve that was causing severe pain across my hip and down my leg, similar to a pinched sciatic nerve.

I was desperate for relief and had heard a colleague, Jasuti Goss, tell of several clients with sciatica she had been able to help, so I decided to ask her to try CranioSacral Therapy on me. I was willing to try anything to get relief from this unbearable pain!

In May I received CranioSacral Therapy from Jasuti, which totally relieved the pain. Since then, I've only had an occasional twinge, but no recurrence of the intense pain and immobility that I had prior to CranioSacral Therapy. I can now do heavy lifting and move objects without triggering another pain episode.

Thanks to CranioSacral Therapy, I am able to continue my work as a massage therapist. I am so grateful that I decided to let Jasuti try to help me. I hope others will decide to try CranioSacral Therapy and not give up hope on having a healthy and full life. There may be hope for them also.

Myra Robison, NCMT
Submitted by Jasuti Goss, NCMT
Anderson, Indiana
CranioSacral Therapy Practitioner since 1998

Inner Physician Says No to Jaw Surgery

Anna, a woman in her late fifties, was referred to me with severe headaches along with jaw, neck, and hip pain. She had been wearing braces on her teeth for a couple of years and was due to be in them for another four years or so. Even then, she was told, she would possibly need jaw surgery.

I began to introduce CranioSacral Therapy to her. Initial general balancing, particularly to her maxilla and zygomas, provided relief from her headaches. She was finally able to get a good night's sleep, which she hadn't been able to do in quite some time.

Following her body's lead, sometimes with the help of her Inner Physician, Anna and I worked together about two or three times a month for a couple of months. We then went to a schedule of once every three to four weeks for several months.

Between visits Anna experienced minimal, if any, head, jaw, neck, or hip pain. Nonetheless, her orthodontist continued to look at surgery. She resisted this idea, though.

At her next appointment, the orthodontist told Anna that she did not need the surgery after all and could get her braces off in a few more months—more than a year and a half earlier than originally suggested. Needless to say, she was quite happy about this new recommendation.

At this writing it has been about two months since Anna got her braces off. I have seen her three times in that period. Her body continues to adjust to not having the braces. After a recent session Anna remarked that she felt "whole."

Maria Scotchell, BA, RMT
Austin, Texas
CranioSacral Therapy Practitioner since 1997

The Lawnmower Meets the Deck

Mira* was referred to me because of her severe headaches and post-concussion syndrome. They had begun a few weeks earlier following an accident while mowing under the deck in her backyard.

She was so engrossed in her activity that she failed to notice the support beam that ran under her deck. Striking her forehead, she was knocked onto her back and lost consciousness for a short time. When she awoke, she had a headache but no other symptoms.

Mira's functioning ability worsened, however, over the course of several weeks. A school secretary for nearly twenty years, she was able to continue doing most of the work tasks with which she was familiar, but she began to have problems with her short-term memory. By Tuesday she would not remember what she had done on Monday and would repeat the same tasks. She was assigned an assistant who prompted her throughout the day to help her complete her job duties.

Mira's headaches gradually increased in frequency and intensity. When a migraine struck, her nausea and visual disturbances made it impossible to work or drive. She would have to call someone to take her home and arrange to have her car picked up. She also began to experience blackouts. During these she would appear normal but have no memory of what she had done for several hours.

I began a 10-Step Protocol on Mira. She went into a deep still point, but when I attempted to lift her frontal bone, it was painful to her. I reasoned that her frontal bone might be jammed under her parietal bones, so I moved to decompress them instead. They released easily. When I returned to the frontal bone, Mira felt an electric charge across her forehead as her frontal bone released. She exclaimed that her head no longer felt so tight. As I continued with

---

*Name changed to protect client confidentiality

the rest of the cranial releases, she reported greater relief.

Mira continued to see me for several weeks and experienced gradual improvement. She returned to work part-time but continued to require CranioSacral Therapy treatments, as her headaches would return. Arcing pointed to areas in her left hip and right shoulder. She remembered two separate accidents where she had injured these areas. Regional tissue releases were done, and she improved enough to return to her former schedule of ten-hour days without experiencing memory loss or migraine.

Peggy Fye, OTR
Kansas City, Kansas
CranioSacral Therapy Practitioner since 1997

Skepticism Turns to Belief as Pain Disappears

My friend's husband was involved in a car-totaling accident and sustained whiplash injuries. He was doctored in the usual way: X-rays, medications, and a cervical collar. His pain was so bad that he couldn't even go to work. It was impossible for him to move his head without severe pain in his neck that ran down his right shoulder.

Every time I saw my friend and she complained about her husband's predicament, I offered to do CranioSacral Therapy on him. They had never heard of CST and were reluctant to try it.

After four weeks of being out of work and enduring insomnia due to his pain, he was ready to try anything. He agreed to let me treat him.

The husband came to my EEG department, and I performed the 10-Step Protocol, paying particular attention to the atlas vertebrae. He fell asleep, completely relaxed, snoring heavily.

When he awoke, he said that he was pain-free for the first time in four weeks! He was amazed. The next day he reported that he had slept like a baby all night and only had a slight ache in his shoulder.

I told him to return for another treatment at the end of the week. On Friday he called and told me that he was just fine and didn't need the appointment. After a couple of days, all discomfort had disappeared.

Barbara Bennett, R EEGT
New Bern, North Carolina
CranioSacral Therapy Practitioner since 2003

The Hope of Feeling Good Again

If you think that you have had too many injuries to be able to return to your old self, think again. Or, if you think the pain is not that bad—you're just a little achy and you can live with it—I must tell you how CranioSacral Therapy made a major difference for me and how wonderful it is not to live with discomfort anymore.

I was familiar with CranioSacral Therapy from treatments given to me by some friends in 1995. When they took the classes they were so excited about it, they worked on me in tandem! It was a wonderful experience. It gave me hope of feeling good again.

I decided to take CranioSacral Therapy classes. When I started using it in my massage therapy business, I wasn't sure if it was making a difference. Then clients started telling me how different they felt and how much they appreciated it.

In October 2002 it was my turn again. I had finally reached a point at which my twenty-plus injuries over the course of twenty-five years had really caught up with me. My body had compromised so much that I was in constant pain, and it was interfering with my ability to work comfortably.

I called Donna Patterson-Kellum, a licensed massage therapist, CranioSacral Therapist, friend, and former co-worker. After six visits of deep emotional and spiritual work, she assessed my needs, and we agreed that I would benefit from a referral for a different depth of work. I believe, however, that I would not have felt safe to move on to treating the physical body if not for the work we did together.

My next stop was Dr. David Young, also a CranioSacral Therapist, who went right to work releasing my abdominal restrictions. We seemed to work well together in helping my body regain its flexibility and use. I experienced some knee swelling as my left thigh learned how to work correctly again. It had been restricted and not of full use for three years. It was amazing how it lost the tonicity and bulk and strength of the entire muscle group. I was having to lift that leg up to get in the car—a small clue that I needed some help getting my body back to working order.

That was December 2002. It is now one and a half years, thirty-seven or so treatments, and another couple of injuries later. I gave David a lot to work on, but I am back! I can walk and enjoy my life without any hesitation. I even squatted and worked in the yard the other day—not a huge task, but one that I had not been able to do for three years. I now have free movement of my pelvis, hip, and knee. I am pain-free. I'm still working on improving the flexibility of my left hip lateral rotation, but I have no pain.

I work in a resort town, so I often see clients for only one visit. Even in that short amount of time I can see what they need in order to enjoy a pain-free life again. I can't refer enough of my clients to CranioSacral Therapy. I know it will help them. I use the International Association of Healthcare Practitioners directory to help them find a practitioner in their area. It fills me with joy to know how wonderful this work is and that my clients will soon experience life anew.

Patrice Tilka, LMT
Cannon Beach, Oregon
CranioSacral Therapy Practitioner since 1996

Sisterly Lesson

In September 2003, I began full-time ministry as a massage therapist at our infirmary for sisters who were retired teachers.

One of the sisters, who was seventy-eight, was having physical challenges following an operation for TMJ. Being that I was also trained in CranioSacral Therapy, I suggested that CST might help. I had recently completed level-two training but hadn't had much opportunity to practice yet. So, while I was convinced that Cranio-Sacral Therapy could make a difference, I wasn't convinced that I was going to be the therapist who would make that difference.

At our first session I felt fairly certain that a fall had contributed to the problem. With my hands on the occiput I began asking a series of questions. I moved my hands to the cheek bones. Sister groaned and said, "Right there! When I was ten I fell off the may-pole and I got hit right there." This body-mind connection allowed us to continue the process of releasing the tight muscles on her whole left side during subsequent sessions. Most recently I worked on releasing the vomer.

(I have subsequently found out that Sister was run over by a truck at the age of five, which resulted in a fractured skull. She was hit in the front teeth when she was twelve. And she was knocked off her bike. No wonder she was having head trauma!)

Some of the changes Sister has experienced include being able to use her left arm again to do simple tasks such as make her bed and reach for things, walk better, and breathe more deeply. Sister can open her mouth wider and swallow better. Before this, she would never think about having a sandwich for lunch, but now she happily enjoys them.

Thanks to Sister's confidence in me, I have since repeated levels one and two of the CranioSacral Therapy coursework, and I look forward to many more wonderful experiences using CST.

Sister Anne Philip, IHM
Immaculata, Pennsylvania
CranioSacral Therapy Practitioner since 2002

If In Doubt, Listen

Marilyn was a forty-three-year-old horse trainer and dressage riding instructor when she came to see me in the spring of 2000. She was referred by her riding friend, a client of mine, who strongly urged Marilyn to "try out this unusual light-touch technique" that seemed to be helping her friend gain more symmetry in her riding.

In rapidly declining health and increasingly frustrated with conventional medicine, Marilyn agreed to try CranioSacral Therapy after hearing about it on several occasions. She hobbled into my clinic, cane in hand and driver in tow.

Marilyn's chief complaints were severe low back pain with radicular symptoms down her left lower extremity, and generalized weakness throughout. Functionally she was unable to sit upright without upper extremity support. She could walk only about a hundred feet using a cane. She was unable to drive. In order to give a riding lesson, she had to lie on her side in the back of a truck and use a microphone for voice projection. All that was on a good day.

Marilyn had an impressive list of medical diagnoses, including degenerative joint disease, permanent impingement of her sciatic nerve, and metabolic myopathy after multiple tests were performed to try and shed light on her mysterious weakening condition.

Her past medical history proved that she was no stranger to injuries. At age six she had fallen hard from a moving wagon onto her sacrum. She had been standing on the edge of the wagon as it rolled out of control down a steep hill. She had experienced difficulty lying on her sacrum ever since. In high school, while going down some rapids on a river trip, she banged her sacrum on a rock. She noticed that the zipper on her jeans could never lie straight after that, a reflection of her pelvic obliquity.

Growing up with horses, Marilyn was bucked off on multiple occasions, again landing on her sacrum. She recalled one occasion when she was thrown off a pony, hit her head on a tree, and went unconscious.

In 1978 she had an inner-tube accident in which she landed on a rock, and her partner landed on top of her. After that episode she began to experience pain on weight-bearing and was able to gain relief with side-lying only. Marilyn took a desk job, which lasted a year. During this time she noticed her left leg weakening.

In 1989 Marilyn experienced another fall off a horse. She sustained a compression fracture of T4-5 [thoracic vertebrae], which further aggravated her lumbar spine and gave rise to hypersensitivity of her thoracic spine. She could no longer ride. After her surgery, she experienced a downward spiral of health.

During this period Marilyn's marriage fell apart, and she relocated to Eden Ranch. She required full-time assistance from her mother for several months to perform all activities of daily living. She became so weak that she could not feed herself. She consulted multiple specialists, went into a pain management program, had physical therapy, sought chiropractic and acupuncture, hired a personal athletic trainer, tried Touch for Health, and followed a strict dietary change.

On my initial evaluation as a physical therapist I found Marilyn to have extremely poor trunkal stability with generalized weakness throughout. She braced her left leg with her cane and tolerated fifty feet of ambulation. On a more subtle level, her cranial rhythm was extremely shallow generally and nonexistent in her pelvic region. She could not lie supine on an air mattress, as this put too much pressure on her occiput and sacrum.

Having only taken the second level of CranioSacral Therapy study at that time, I felt overwhelmed. Where should I begin? I decided to follow the voices of my instructors: If in doubt, do the 10-Step Protocol.

I saw Marilyn once or twice a week for three months before we saw any sign of progress. Significant changes occurred after a successful sacral decompression. Within a year we had exceeded her goal of walking without a cane. Not only was she able to drive herself to the clinic, she was able to get back on a horse.

By the time her insurance coverage ended, our friendship had grown. We began trading services when she was able to resume her life as a riding instructor. She continues to receive CranioSacral Therapy in conjunction with other disciplines I learned from The Upledger Institute.

Today Marilyn has returned to competitive riding, trains young horses, coaches quadrille teams, and rides five or six horses a day. Her energy level exceeds mine. She has regained her sculptured physique and exhibits only minor telltale signs of a rotated pelvis and scoliosis of the spine. I frequently hear her say that Cranio-Sacral Therapy has given her back her life. I need no further reward.

Pat Thummanond, PT
Fresno, California
CranioSacral Therapy Practitioner since 1993

Something Good from Something Bad

On Chinese New Year, February 1, 2003, I herniated a disc in my neck (C6-C7). It was an unusual accident. My boyfriend and I were just fooling around, wrestling, and I flipped over and landed wrong. I heard a crunch and knew it was not good.

A couple of days later I went to see my chiropractor, who told me that she thought I would be okay and to just take it easy for a while. Well, my interpretation of taking it easy was not the same as hers, and I really overdid it. I continued to lift weights, swim, and run just as usual. The injury worsened. It got so bad that I had difficulty working at the computer, playing the piano and fiddle, or lifting anything without my right hand and arm causing me extreme pain and numbness.

I went back to my chiropractor, who told me to stop doing everything. She adjusted me and gave me a neck brace to wear. I was very unhappy.

A few months earlier I had signed up for a massage therapy class as an adjunct to my nursing profession. I was looking forward to getting to do some hands-on work with people to help them feel better. Here I was instead, in pain myself and unable to do anything but yoga.

By "chance," when I was in getting acupuncture from my regular medical doctor, I saw a coupon for a free CranioSacral Therapy session with a local physical therapist. I thought it couldn't hurt to try, as I was very frustrated with my healing timeline.

The night after my first session, I had a very intense Somato-Emotional Release. I cried harder than I ever had before, and afterwards I felt so good. I continued to see this therapist once a week for about a month with continued healing results, both physical and emotional.

Because CranioSacral Therapy had helped me so much, I decided to take the entry-level course instead of the massage class. It was one of the best decisions I ever made. I share it with everyone I meet, and I work on anyone who is open to it. I just purchased a portable massage table in order to work on people in their homes. I use CST with Reiki, which makes for a very healing combination.

The lesson for me in all this is that even when something happens to me that looks bad, it can always turn into something good. My next dream is to go to Florida and experience CranioSacral Therapy with the dolphins!

Dee Vogel, RN
Placerville, California
CranioSacral Therapy Practitioner since 2003

"The Headache Chaser"

✿ I took my first CranioSacral Therapy (CST) class in the summer of 2003. Returning to the massage therapy school where I teach, I encountered two students who were experiencing terrible migraine headaches and had been for nearly four days. One lady was going to drop out of school because it was just too difficult and painful to attend class.

Excited to try my newly learned skill, I brought each of them into my classroom one at a time during the hands-on lab period. It ended up being not only me and these two ladies, but nearly sixteen other students who were curious to see what CranioSacral Therapy was about. They wanted to know how something so gentle, which looked as if I did nothing, could help them.

The first lady got instant, total relief. The second got relief from more than half the pain and all the visual issues. The next day the second lady asked for another treatment. By the end she had complete relief from all the pain.

This encounter with CST made believers of me, the two ladies, and most of the school body. Eight students and two teachers even signed up to learn CranioSacral Therapy after that!

Word is now out at school that I am the headache chaser. It has been the single most effective method of treatment I have ever learned. I personally want to thank Dr. Upledger for his magnificent contributions to the welfare and betterment of humankind.

Andrea K. Collier, CMT
Templeton, Pennsylvania
CranioSacral Therapy Practitioner since 2003

Headaches and Dizziness Sent Packing with CST

A friend of mine for many years asked me if CranioSacral Therapy (CST) might help her with her dizzy spells. Whenever she turned her head to do head and neck exercises, she would become dizzy and unable to continue. The dizziness distressed her at other times, too, but this seemed to trouble her the most.

I was a fairly green CST beginner at the time, and my friend would be my first 10-Step Protocol client. Although I had done massage for twenty years and am a certified rehabilitation registered nurse, neither of these skills are remotely like CST. So in response to my friend's question, I quoted Dr. Upledger, who said he didn't know what conditions couldn't be helped by Cranio-Sacral Therapy, and that he trusted the techniques.

I followed the steps of the protocol. She was thrilled afterward to be able to once again do her head and neck exercises and to meditate. I asked her to let me know how long the effects lasted.

My friend reported back that she did not have any dizziness for a month. She returned a few more times over the next few months for repeat sessions. We were both very pleased.

An elderly lady I had recently met was suffering from constant headaches after an auto accident. She had tried a variety of medications and mainstream medical approaches, but nothing was helping. I offered to give her a free session just to see if CranioSacral Therapy might be of benefit.

I did the 10-Step Protocol on this woman. When she sat up from the table she began to smile and nearly jumped up and down with happiness. Her headache was gone at last—and it has stayed gone.

Another friend of mine suffered from chronic migraines, sometimes twice a week, for most of her life. She consented to let me practice on her for an upcoming CranioSacral Therapy seminar I was preparing for.

I wasn't sure if CST would help, because this friend generally didn't go in for things like bodywork or visualization or other alternative modalities. I was just pleased that she was willing to give this a try. We chatted during the session, and when it was done we went to dinner and a movie.

A few days later my friend called and informed me that she hadn't had any headaches and was happy about that. Over a month went by, and she was still headache-free. Since nothing else had changed in her habits, she had to admit that CST had done the job.

I like the fact that I do not have to apply pounds of pressure to do CranioSacral Therapy; the weight of a nickel is plenty. I also like conversing with the client's Inner Physician to negotiate relief via intention. The power of intention is profound, as are the CST techniques and the feather-light touch. Thanks for sharing the knowledge and for making the seminars so comfortable and efficient.

Leslie Aguillard, RN, CRRN
Denver, Colorado
CranioSacral Therapy Practitioner since 1999

Thirty Years of Pain Come to an End

In early 2002 I worked on a very sweet woman named Margi, who had gone through a car windshield in 1972. In a coma for three months, she had awakened to find her face reconstructed. Ever since, she had experienced daily headaches that ranged in intensity from bad to almost debilitating.

At the beginning of the CranioSacral Therapy session, she demonstrated a very weak and erratic rhythm. The bones were all very jammed together. Movement ranged from barely perceptible to basically none at all. I worked for an hour doing a basic CST protocol.

As I went from step to step, Margi's bones began to loosen. When I did the release using the ears, there was a sudden, intense movement. Her headache stopped. She was thrilled.

After a few weeks, Margi's headache began to come back, but only a little. She came in and we did another CST session. About four weeks after that, when her headaches began again, she came in for a third session.

I now see Margi every few months, usually in social situations. She occasionally has headaches "like other people," as she puts it, but has never again had the headaches with which she lived for thirty years.

Connie Wehmeyer, LMT
Warwick, New York
CranioSacral Therapy Practitioner since 1998

I Can See Clearly Now the Pain Is Gone

❁ I was working for some physical therapists on the north side of Houston. They worked in one room and I, a massage therapist, worked in a separate room in the back. One morning a middle-aged woman walked in and proceeded to tell me that I was her last hope. She informed me that if I could not help her, she was going to commit suicide.

About a year earlier, she had been watching a soccer game when a stray ball hit her on the side of the head. About two weeks later she started getting headaches, her vision blurred, and her teeth and jaw structure no longer fit properly. She began wearing thick glasses and a mouth guard all the time. The worsening state left her in excruciating pain 24/7.

The woman told me that she had seen dozens of doctors, therapists, and specialists. She had taken every type of test recommended with absolutely no results. She also had tried every kind of pain medication with no relief.

Being a CranioSacral Therapist trained to look at the body in different ways, I told her that I might have a solution to her dilemma. I asked her to lie down face up, and I put my hands on her head very lightly. What I felt was truly amazing. Her temporal bones, which should move in unison, were almost one hundred eighty degrees out of phase.

I asked her to remove her glasses and look up at the ceiling. She let me know that everything was totally blurred. As I readjusted her temporal bones, reestablishing a proper phase relationship, her vision started correcting and clearing. Within seconds her vision returned to what it had been before the accident, and she no longer needed her glasses to see.

I started working on the other areas of the skull. Within forty-five minutes she was totally out of pain; her headaches were completely gone; and her teeth and jaw fit perfectly. Needless to say, this woman was thrilled and overjoyed.

Thank you, Dr. John Upledger, for sharing your knowledge and the wonderful technique we all know and love as CranioSacral Therapy.

Danny D. Dore, RMT
Houston, Texas
CranioSacral Therapy Practitioner since 1993

Breaking the Cycle of Prescription Drugs

❀ I have been a licensed massage therapist for five years. I took my first CranioSacral Therapy (CST) class one month after taking the Ohio State Medical Board exam for licensure. I knew that I wanted CST to be the focus of my bodywork practice. The following is a testimonial from one of my clients at my hospital-based Holistic Health Center practice.

"Two years ago I had colon cancer surgery and since then have had periodic abdominal spasms, which were attributed to the healing process. Last fall, the spasms became constant and unbearable. Doctors ruled out the return of cancer, hernias, irritable bowel syndrome, and reproductive problems. I was on six different pharmaceuticals and was extremely frustrated.

"The week of Thanksgiving, I attended a special-education conference that included workshops on ADHD and autism. A workshop on autism specifically addressed CranioSacral Therapy and its benefits. Massage therapy and its benefits were also discussed in several workshops, including one on stress management. When I arrived home later that day and was going through my mail, I discovered the latest edition of *Healthy Neighbors,* which described the various services offered by the Holistic Health Center.

"The next day I made an appointment for a sixty-minute total-body massage. The therapist took my complete medical history and asked me questions about my health, job, family, and habits before beginning. The therapist taught me a massage technique that I could use myself to alleviate some of the discomfort I was experiencing in the abdominal region.

"Afterward, she discussed what she had found during the massage and recommended various therapies that could benefit me. She also said that she thought another therapist trained in CST could give me more or better relief than she could. I made an appointment for a ninety-minute session two weeks later.

"After the first CST session, I was able to reduce the amount of medications I was taking. After the second visit, I was only taking one medication at bedtime. By the third, I was not taking anything at all for the abdominal spasms.

"I continue to use the massage techniques I was shown, and only use one medication at bedtime on rare occasions when I have overestimated my recovery process.

"I think the most amazing thing that has occurred is the amount of energy I have begun to have since beginning CST. Friends and family members constantly comment on my new demeanor. They say I seem happier and healthier than I have in a long time. I personally feel more able to tolerate stress. And instead of having to rest because I am tired or in pain, I have more energy to do things with my family.

"The most surreal thing is the amount of toxins my body puts out after each therapy session. For several days following a treatment, my husband comments on the odors that emanate from my body—predominantly anesthesia!"

Judy Molique, LMT
Cincinnati, Ohio
CranioSacral Therapy Practitioner since 2000

Magical Journey

✿ In 1994 I was traveling in Oaxaca, Mexico, with a friend. I had just spent three months studying Spanish at the University of Queretaro and was living with a host family. My friend and I decided to travel for two weeks before returning home to the United States. It was a hot summer day and we had just gotten off an eight-hour bus ride. We checked into a hotel a few blocks from the beach, and I decided to go for a swim in the ocean. It was beautiful and the water was warm. I decided to do a little body surfing and caught a few waves into shore.

To my dismay, the last wave I rode that day swept me away with it. As I crashed back on shore, I felt my entire body crunch. The strength of the ocean drove me into the earth, cracking my spine, twisting and turning me, and eventually spitting me back out. The result was a shattered humerus, fractured scapula, and a fractured clavicle on my right side, plus massive bruising and spinal misalignments.

A long, agonizing, two-day bus ride took me to hospitals in Mexico, where I was informed of the fractures. All they could offer me, though, were painkillers and advice to go back to the States. I caught a flight home to a hospital that had the technology to do a CAT scan.

The specialist told me that the fractures were being held in place by my muscles, which fortunately had not torn. They said they could do surgery but were not sure if it would help matters. My other option was to just put an immobilizer on my arm and allow my body to heal it on its own. I chose option two. I did not want to go under the knife.

I called around to see if any of my friends had any ideas for therapy. As fate would have it, I landed in the very loving, healing hands of a physical therapist specializing in CranioSacral Therapy (CST). The person who referred me said that he could not explain what she did; he just knew it had really helped him to resolve some shoulder pain that he was having.

For months I went once a week for CranioSacral Therapy. At times the healing was dramatic, and at other times miraculous. I started out with my shoulder swollen and purple; I looked like a football player on one side. I was in so much pain I could barely walk. I could not sleep and was crying constantly.

After my first session I remember having a profound sense of hope return to me. Prior to that I did not have the use of my arm; I could not move it or lift it. Someone had to help me shower and change my clothes. I kept my arm in an immobilizer whenever I could to prevent it from dislocating due to its own weight.

The first change I noticed was periods without pain. Then I began to regain use of my arm. Before this I had to use my left hand to shift gears in the car. Slowly I was able to do it with my right arm again.

I asked so many questions during my sessions that my therapist offered to lend me some books to read on CranioSacral Therapy. I went through some profound emotional releases on her table as I relived the trauma. Somehow that experience released the fear out of my body so that I could jump to a higher level of peace and comfort within myself. I was able to receive the gift of the experience.

I felt the therapist cultivating my strength. She inspired my healing on so many levels. My arm and my spirit were transformed within months. I felt like a bird with a mended broken wing that could fly again. My entire world was changing for the better.

Very quickly I found my life revolving around CranioSacral Therapy. I returned to school to complete my bachelor's degree in art, but was so longing to study CST that I found a way to complete my last two terms at the University doing an independent study as an apprentice with my physical therapist.

I was so in love with the work that I felt the desire pushing me to go back to college to get a license in order to do the work professionally. I also started to study the work formally through The Upledger Institute.

I have seen a wide variety of pain and discomfort, and I am always impressed at the numerous ways CranioSacral Therapy can help to ease peoples' experiences into healing ones—my own experiences included. I now have full range of motion in my right arm and shoulder. I can dance, swim, raft, and carry a backpack in the wilderness for days.

I am forever grateful to my first mentor who helped me to heal myself so that I could assist others in their healing. From my firsthand experience of healing, I realize that anything is possible, and the journey is a magical one.

Heather Navarrete-Linnemeyer, BA, LMT, CST-D
Grants Pass, Oregon
CranioSacral Therapist since 1995

CST Brings Healing Through Seasons of Life

It all started quite unexpectedly. There was a lot of sadness, anger, and tension in my life that year. The company where I had worked for more than twenty years changed hands, and I was without a job. My mother passed away, and I had to clean out a house that our family had lived in for fifty years. It felt like I died, too, and was clearing out my own life. Only a few months later, my husband's parents became very sick and we went to Los Angeles to help out.

Browsing in a book store one day, I came across a flyer for a "relaxing and nurturing massage." I could certainly use that, I thought. I made an appointment, and that's when I first met James. He took one look at me and said, "Would you like to try something different?" Well, I'm usually game for a new adventure, and he looked trustworthy, so I agreed.

"Take off your shoes and let me help you onto the massage table," James said. He proceeded to place his hands gently on my body, without any rubbing or massaging, and just held them there quietly for a while. My eyes closed. Then he moved his hands here and there, and then around my head.

This was one hour of bliss. I seemed to travel through the universe, passing the stars along the way. I was slightly awake, enough to know that someone was in the room and to feel warm hands moving from place to place. It was my first hour of many to come of CranioSacral Therapy (CST).

I quickly learned that my favorite experience was when James put his hands on my head. Almost instantly I forgot all my daily aggravations and entered the world of carefree. This was soon followed by visions, like dreams. Our work together progressed, and soon I was talking with body parts and listening to events that had happened during my life—unpleasant memories that had become stored in my body and had manifested in various chronic aches and pains. Boy, did I have a lot of baggage to unload!

Although releasing the emotional issues was sometimes very difficult, very difficult indeed, my CST sessions became the highlight of my week, and I looked forward to them. Each one was different. Each was an adventure.

I became so intrigued with this form of healing that I went to learn how to do it myself. I've since added CST to other forms of healing I had learned. Now that I'm back home in Israel, I've started to expose people here to the wonders of CST. I love being a part of someone's healing process.

For me, the healing work of CranioSacral Therapy is so amazing. When I lost my job as a secretary, I knew that I didn't want to work in an office again. I didn't know what I would do next. CST relieved my tensions, healed old emotional wounds, fixed chronic aches and pains, and got me started on a new career path, as well.

I still wanted to continue with my own personal journey, so I searched for another CranioSacral Therapist close to home and finally found Efraim. I am currently suffering from symptoms of a major disease, and we've been working at getting to the core of why this has appeared at this time of my life and what I'm supposed to learn from it. Efraim's background is medicine, so I'm taking advantage of that knowledge, too. He's become a great partner to work with. This story doesn't have an ending yet; I hope it will be a happy one.

Judith Lebowitz-Cohn
Jerusalem, Israel
CranioSacral Therapy Practitioner since 2002

Surrendering to the Touch

My mom Rita called me after a serious spinout. A bright, healthy, strong, seventy-one-year-old redheaded Irish woman, she had been reeling with vertigo for two days. Though she wanted my help, she had some issues with trusting anyone, including me, to touch the back of her neck. I went over to her condo anyway, table in tow, around eleven-thirty that night.

I worked the CranioSacral Therapy protocol slowly. Within an hour, Mom's head popped almost as loudly as bubblegum. She lay there about thirty minutes and then slowly sat up. She wept in my arms, feeling a tremendous amount of surrender and absolution.

It's been over a year now, and Mom has never had another dizzy spell. She says that night saved her life in a way not too many people would understand. I thought you all might.

Maryanne Natale-Royal
Dunedin, Florida
CranioSacral Therapy Practitioner since 2001

A New Release on Life

In 1993 Katy was rear-ended in an automobile accident involving the force of two cars. She suffered two herniated discs. A chiropractor she went to suggested that she visit a neurosurgeon, who ended up removing one disc and fusing two others. She continued working with the chiropractor and a physical therapist after the surgery.

As Katy was improving from this accident, she was involved in yet another one in 1998. Again she was rear-ended, and again she worked with her chiropractor. The neurosurgeon determined that further surgery on the remaining herniated disc would not help at this time.

Suffering from severe headaches and nausea, Katy was referred to a special physical therapist who worked with her intensely twice a week. She had to travel one hour each way for these treatments. Still she continued to suffer from extreme headaches. Eventually her chiropractor put her in a padded metal neck brace with a chin support, which she was supposed to wear sixteen hours a day to get the headache level down.

Desperate to get out of the brace, Katy visited an acupuncturist. She had a severe reaction, however, that left her in bed with the most severe migraine-like headache and nausea she had ever experienced. Her chiropractor and the acupuncturist were able to suggest treatments to get the reaction to end.

Katy had been wearing the neck brace for two and a half years when she was referred to me in 2001. Worried that she might have to wear this the rest of her life, her main goal was to get out of the brace. If she took it off, the headaches and nausea were unbearable.

The first time I saw Katy, very early on in my CranioSacral Therapy practice, I started with the 10-Step Protocol. I spent the entire hour on the pelvic and diaphragmatic releases. The second time, I continued with the thoracic region and cranial base. Finally, the third time, I worked intently on each of the vertebrae. The CV-3 took about twenty-five minutes to unwind and finally resolve. After completing the entire spine, I finished up with the cranial bones and a still point.

After the third treatment Katy decided to try and go without the neck brace. It worked! The headaches were lessened so much that she was able to go without the brace that she had worn for two and a half years. She could now do laundry, make dinner, and wash the kitchen floor. Soon after this, her first grandbaby was born, and she was able to enjoy and hold the infant without pain.

Following up with Katy three years later, I found out that she was still without the brace and her headache level remained low. She even occasionally experienced times when there was no pain at all.

Thanks, Katy, for making a believer out of me.

Kristen Murphy
Santa Monica, California
CranioSacral Therapy Practitioner since 1999

CranioSacral Therapy on the Road in India

❁ The bus is starting to move. We are finally on our way to fulfill our Buddhist pilgrimage. There are about forty of us from the United States, Puerto Rico, Mongolia, Russia, and India. Among our Indian companions are Buddhist monks, a nun, and a young girl with a beautiful smile from Tibet, two nuns from Bhutan, and five from Nepal, including our bus driver and cook. The nuns and monks all wear the same deep red robes and their heads are shaved. Along with all this human cargo, the bus is carrying cartons of water, luggage, ritual objects such as long horns and drums, and cases of candles.

It becomes a common sight to see the cows meandering down the road, unrestrained amidst bicycles, cars, ox carts, trucks and bus traffic. Horns blow continuously, which is considered polite driving there; it lets everyone know that the vehicle is coming. Fields alternate with shanties and larger buildings lining the road. Everything is covered by dust, and whenever our air-conditioned bus door opens or a window is cracked, we breathe it in. We crawl along the barely paved road, dodging the other vehicles and bumping over continuous potholes.

Our pilgrimage starts out from Sarnath, the city where Buddha gave his first teaching after he became enlightened. We are headed for Shravasti, where Buddha lived for twenty-five summers teaching, performing miracles, and overseeing a monastery with more than a hundred monks.

Our group has been supporting the building of a stupa, or shrine, in Shravasti. The stupa is a replica of one built by Buddha twenty-five hundred years earlier in the same spot but destroyed long ago. The building of the new stupa is complete, and the purpose of our pilgrimage is its consecration and ceremonial opening to the public. It is named The Miracle Stupa for World Peace, and its interior shrine room can hold more than one hundred people.

We ride for about four hours before stopping for lunch at a roadside restaurant. One of the Bhutanese nuns, who looks to be about nineteen years old, complains of a migraine. Her head hurts along the frontal area, and she is having trouble with her eyes. I ask her to sit at one of the outdoor tables.

We've been traveling on a main highway that, in the United States, would be considered the worst of country roads. Barely wide enough for two vehicles, it is jammed with trucks, buses, bicycles, rickshaws, ox carts, pedestrians, school children, cars, cows, dogs, goats, donkeys, and monkeys. It is bumpy and dusty. The straw shacks and brick houses on the side of the road wear layers of dust.

The nun, Ani Konchok Yangchen, sits at a table and I stand behind her. Her sphenoid is displaced superior with a severe left anterior strain. Her left temporal is completely jammed, and her right is almost as bad. I can place my thumbs on her sphenoid at the temple area, and my little fingers can reach the occiput. I can feel the strain quite clearly. I asked her inner wisdom what it would like me to do.

The sphenoid begins to unlock and move cautiously in a crooked cranial rhythm. I go along for the ride. As it moves in flexion, I encourage it off its stuck position on the sphenobasilar synchondrosis. It responds with increased amplitude and begins to move more freely. I follow and encourage. I feel it shift.

After some time, I move to the temporals. In the standing position, I access them with the tips of my fingers as if working in the spokes of a wheel. Again, I ask what they want. They immediately go out of sync, and I feel like I am shaking the rust out of the joints.

The amplitude improves and the temporals come back into sync. They begin moving more freely. The young nun smiles and says she is starting to feel better. I finish by opening her lymph pathways at the clavicles and neck.

Someone gives her a bottle of water, and I tell her to drink it all right away. Then, we're back in the bus bumping along rather quickly. I'm thinking that it would truly take a miracle for anyone to get rid of a migraine under these conditions.

The monks tell us that we have almost reached the stupa, but it turns out to be another two to three hours. The nun is sitting far behind me, and I can't see her to check on how she's doing. I try to sleep.

The monks begin singing deep-throated chanting prayers, and we catch our first sight of The Miracle Stupa for World Peace. It's so white! And so big! Rising about ninety feet, its white body, rainbow-colored cylindrical top, and multi-colored prayer flags stand out impressively against the gray evening sky.

We pour out of the bus, overcome with the awe of The Miracle Stupa's beauty. We're all chattering, laughing, and hugging each other. I see Ani Konchok. She is all smiles.

"Much better," she calls out to me in her simple English. "All better. I feel good."

Elizabeth Pasquale, LMT, CST
Ossining, New York
CranioSacral Therapy Practitioner since 1998

Migraine Victim Is Freed

❀ I began my massage therapy career in March of 1999 full of enthusiasm, ready to "fix" the world. In my quest for further knowledge, I immediately signed up for a CranioSacral Therapy class taught by The Upledger Institute.

At first, most of my therapy work consisted of Swedish massage. I was working at the time in a couple of salons and building a client base. Shortly after I struck out on my own, one of my female clients asked me about CranioSacral Therapy. She had read about it in a newsletter I sent out.

This client's concern was not for herself but for her son's girl-friend Jamie.* She informed me that Jamie was experiencing throwing-up kinds of migraines on a weekly basis. I assured my client that CranioSacral Therapy would do no harm to the girl. After our discussion it was agreed that Jamie would come in for a session.

I told the young lady—I believe she was twenty-one—that I wanted her to be comfortable. All she needed to do was kick off her shoes, lie on her back, and I would do the rest. The session began with her wondering: What is he doing with this gentle touch?

As I began to lay my hands above and below her to release the pelvis, I asked her what she was feeling. Jamie replied that she could feel me moving my hands in a circular motion. That's when I sur-prised her by letting her know that I was only following her lead. She was doing the moving. "Wow!" she said in total amazement.

As the session went on, nothing really spectacular happened until I got up around Jamie's neck. All of a sudden her whole body jumped. It startled me, as well as her. When I asked her if she was all right, she replied, "This is so cool!"

After the session she told her boyfriend's mother what had hap-pened. She said that she felt very, very relaxed, as though she had

---

*Name changed to protect client confidentiality

had many hours of sleep.

After that session, Jamie's migraines diminished to an occasional rather than weekly basis. After about two years she came back for a good Swedish massage. We talked about migraines, but for the most part, that one eighty-minute session of CranioSacral Therapy was all it had taken to get her system up and running smoothly again.

Don M. Williams, RMT
Arlington, Texas
CranioSacral Therapy Practitioner since 1999

"My Friends Would Think I'm Crazy"

❀ I had always pictured meat cutters to be tall and burly, so I was surprised to hear that it was what my next patient did for a living. John was a little man with well-developed muscles who came to see me because he had received a gift certificate for a massage. He had never had one before and was very hesitant coming into the session.

I had just returned from my first CranioSacral Therapy class and was taking every opportunity I could to practice. I now made it a habit to start every session by trying to get information from the tissues, learning to listen.

To my surprise John's left hand began to shake as soon as I touched his head. I watched his hand, feeling sorry that the poor man was so nervous. Then I realized that only his left hand was shaking. It began to move laterally away from his body, then up toward the ceiling.

John was paying attention and looking up at me. Finally he asked how I could possibly move his arm by touching his head—the dreaded question when you are starting a new therapy, are unsure of yourself, and are second-guessing whether you are actually feeling what you think you are feeling. At least the movement was visible.

John's arm continued to move until it reached the level of his shoulder. Then it stopped, shook, and continued to move above his head, stretching out next to my body as I sat at the head of the table.

John was sobbing as he told me that he had been unable to raise his left arm above his head for the past six years, ever since he had overextended and torn the muscles in his rotator cuff as he attempted to throw a side of beef into the grinder. Though the injury had been surgically repaired and he had received plenty of physical therapy, he had been unable to lift his arm beyond shoulder level since the accident. Looking up at me, he yelled that he couldn't possibly be doing this, that it was not a possible position for his arm—all this as his arm remained stretched out and trembling above his head. Slowly the arm began its journey back to its original position.

John was still crying when I began the massage that he had come in for. He began telling me his story, how he hadn't cried since he was six years old. He was trying to convince me that he had a good life—a good marriage, nice kids, a job he liked—and thus had no reason to cry. He was embarrassed to be so wimpy. He had grown up with a father who had told him that if he cried, he would for sure give him a reason to.

On his way out, John asked if he could give me a hug. He said, "I have no idea what happened in there, how you did what you did to me, but I thank you for that experience. I hope you understand, though, that I will never tell a soul what I experienced, because my friends would think I am crazy."

Ilona E. Trommler, LMT
Westlake, Ohio
CranioSacral Therapy Practitioner since 1998

Desperation

✻ The day I arrived at The Upledger Institute HealthPlex clinic for an Intensive Program in July 2004 was my first step in returning "home" to my true self. What gave me the hope and determination to pursue this course was a man in his thirties who had been in a motorcycle accident.

A patient in the program like me, he said, "I credit CranioSacral Therapy with ninety percent of my recovery." He'd been told by doctors that he would be permanently paralyzed from the neck down. He was now walking with a limp, but he was walking all the same!

I had come in desperation. I was angry, too. Pain does that to you. I had tried everything possible, from homeopathy to meditation to herbs and diet. This was my last hope.

To be perfectly honest, I was hoping on the way to the clinic that the plane would crash and I wouldn't have to live with this agony any longer. Everything I tried had given some temporary relief, but the awful pain would always come back.

For twenty-four years I lived in severe, chronic pelvic pain. This began with the birth of my second child and the use of a rigid arc-spring diaphragm. The muscle between the rectum and vagina had been ripped entirely away. After five months of tests, exams, and basically being told I was crazy, a laparoscopy answered the question. The next day the muscle was reattached and I was ecstatic.

Then I developed peritonitis. My belly blew up like a balloon and pus poured from my umbilicus. This created adhesions (sticky scar tissue) that covered all my organs. Over the next fifteen months I had five more surgeries to basically remove the adhesions. These also included scraping of the coccyx and a partial hysterectomy (left ovary remained).

The abdominal surgeries always took four hours, because it took that long to cut through the adhesions to find my organs. After one of the surgeries, my bowel collapsed. A tube attached to a bag of mercury was shoved down my nose into the intestine until the obstruction was opened. If this hadn't succeeded I would have needed another abdominal surgery to open the obstruction.

We moved from Michigan to North Carolina in 1980. I was always in pain. Different holistic modalities kept me existing. On seeing a homeopathic doctor, he discovered a large ovarian cyst in my pelvis. The gynecologist recommended surgery.

Again it took four hours to cut through the adhesions and find the cyst, which was the size of a grapefruit. It was months before I could even stand. Three years later came reconstruction surgery. There was some relief, then the pain always returned.

As a lactation consultant, helping mothers and their babies with breastfeeding, I had referred several babies to a local CranioSacral Therapist with good results. Specifically, their severe crying had resolved.

I decided to pursue this therapy for myself. After receiving some temporary relief with CranioSacral Therapy, I decided to take a class.

Here I was now, a year later, in the Intensive Program.

Almost immediately I felt safe. I realized that it wasn't my responsibility to deal with the pain. Over the course of the program I just opened and accepted.

I returned to the clinic several times after that first Intensive Program, and I continue to receive CranioSacral Therapy on a regular basis, along with Visceral Manipulation and Lymph Drainage Therapy. Because of this, I can now say that I am pain-free, and I am continuing to heal. This experience of getting better and becoming more alive each day is very addicting.

Rosemary Kolasa, RD, MPH, IBCLC
Durham, North Carolina
CranioSacral Therapy Practitioner since 2003

Niagara 911

It was August of 2003. I was just minding my own business, vacationing amidst an array of souvenirs in an outlook tower high over Niagara Falls, when I noticed an elderly lady slouching against the glass observation wall. My hands wanted to touch her, but I restrained myself, not wanting to embarrass my sister and her friend Laurie, a registered nurse. As we passed by, I had second thoughts and started to say, "Laurie, do you mind if we take a moment to help?" By the time I turned back, the lady had already lost consciousness.

Laurie immediately began taking the lady's pulse. She did not tell me at the time that her vitals were quickly fading. I used Dr. Upledger's arcing technique and said to Laurie, "She wants me to work on her right arm." Laurie repeated, saying, "She wants you to work on her right arm" in a tone that I interpreted as: "Yeah, right, this lady wants you to work on her right arm when her heart is fading. And, in her condition, you're expecting me to believe that she could ask you for anything."

I was so relieved that Laurie was there, taking over the medical issues, asking someone to call 911, taking the lady's pulse, determining that oxygen would be helpful. What she couldn't determine, and was eager to know, was the lady's blood pressure. Laurie said to me, "I do this stuff all the time, but this is so different. I usually work in a room where I have all the equipment I need."

As Laurie continued to try to monitor the lady's condition, I continued to let my hands lead me in treatment. Laurie noticed and commented that the woman was making marked improvements as I worked.

When a nearby vendor finally found an old oxygen tank, Laurie struggled to quickly learn how to use the dated machine. She put the yellowed mask on the lady's face, still wishing that there could be a way to take the woman's blood pressure.

By the time the rescue workers arrived and got to us, the woman was conscious and appeared almost normal. I urged Laurie to let the paramedics know, in whatever medical terms would be most convincing, that the lady needed further observation. Her elderly husband, however, insisted that she was fine. He believed she had just been resting for a moment, and he could take her home.

That evening, I overheard Laurie on her cell phone. She was talking to her mother, the director of nurses in a very well-known hospital in our region. It sounded as though Laurie believed that the woman would not have survived without "whatever it was" I was doing.

It was then that I was deeply awed by all that had happened that morning. A registered nurse had brought the expertise of Western medicine. A CranioSacral Therapist had listened and responded to the directives of the lady's Inner Physician. And my sister, a member of a religious order of women, had definitely supported all of us with the grace and power of prayer.

Catherine L. Schneider, MA, LMT
Toledo, Ohio
CranioSacral Therapy Practitioner since 1998

"This CST Really Works!"

✿ I had just finished my first CranioSacral Therapy (CST) class and was interested in getting my hands on people to try out my new skill. I put up a sign offering CST sessions at the local massage school that I had attended six months earlier. I received a phone call about a week later from a student who had just taken a brief introductory class in CST and was really interested in taking the level-one course in a few months.

Debra was a forty-seven-year-old female nurse studying to become a licensed massage therapist in Florida. She came to me with a chronically sore shoulder and stiff neck. While the problem wasn't really hindering her, she had had no success in getting rid of it, either.

Debra had been in an accident years before while nursing. She had been trying to help a patient move from the bed to a wheelchair when the patient's leg gave out. In reaching to grab the patient before he went crashing to the floor, she badly pulled her shoulder and hurt her neck.

I told her that I would do my best, and we would see how she felt. The standard 10-Step Protocol lasted just about an hour, and afterwards she said she felt better. I admit to feeling a bit discouraged at the time that she was still feeling the problem at all. As a massage therapist, I knew that most people feel better after getting worked on.

I didn't hear from Debra for about five months. Then one day she stopped by to tell me what had happened after her Cranio-Sacral Therapy session. The day after she had been in extreme pain. She had even considered calling to yell at me, even though I had explained that her body would have to accept this new change and that she might feel some "shifts" during the next few days that followed.

By the second day, less than forty-eight hours post-treatment,

Debra was pain-free, and any restrictions she had had from the injury were completely gone. She has yet to have the pain return and has decided to pursue CST further in her own practice.

Needless to say, this story has been a huge motivational factor for me in pursuing CranioSacral Therapy work, and it has become a blessing for my practice.

Michele Mathiesen, LMT, NMT
Sarasota, Florida
CranioSacral Therapy Practitioner since 2003

Spontaneous Remission

✿ "You fixed my headaches!" the woman exclaimed as she hobbled over and hugged me. At first I thought she had confused me with another therapist. It turned out that I had seen her as a CranioSacral Therapy (CST) client six weeks prior to the party we were both now attending.

Not recalling her situation, I asked her what she was referring to. For thirty years she had been treated for persistent, severe headaches. In order to receive the pain pills she needed, she was periodically required to undergo medical tests, because the physical consequences of their long-term use were so grave. Even then she was allowed only a few pills a month.

She indicated that she had begun having these headaches in her early twenties, and the pain was often extremely severe. In fact, she had planned to check herself into the hospital for treatment right after our appointment. Following her CST session, however, her head had not hurt at all, and her severe pain had not returned.

She hobbled that evening because she had a cast on her leg from an athletic injury sustained a few days prior. Following this injury she had experienced her first headache in more than five weeks. It did not require the strong medication she had previously taken, and it had subsided within twenty-four hours.

When I got to my office the next day, I looked over my notes from her visit. She had not mentioned a health problem of any type during our interview or on the intake form. She was a bodywork regular and routinely received chiropractic care, CranioSacral Therapy, and massage from other therapists.

The single CranioSacral Therapy session I performed was routine and unremarkable, except for the removal of multiple energy cysts. Once these were cleared, I had been able to obtain a complete pelvic floor diaphragm release. Her tissues had been really easy to work with.

During her session, she had indicated that she did not like emotional expression during bodywork, although she completed a SomatoEmotional Release easily as she recalled an incident that occurred on the playground in elementary school. With a mixture of laughter and tears, she recalled being choked by a classmate who had grabbed her school tie while trying to keep her from recovering a ball. This memory popped up as I was releasing the tissue of her cervical spine and throat. She had not expressed any discomfort or embarrassment during or after the process.

I am often completely amazed at how basic CranioSacral Therapy skills applied as taught can produce immediate health restoration. In class, the instructors say, "Evaluate and treat what you find. Leave the results up to the client and the Inner Physician." Very true, very wise.

Doris Weiner, RMT
Plano, Texas
CranioSacral Therapy Practitioner since 2000

From Hobbies to Horses, Pain-Free

❀ Nola, age fifty-eight, first came to see me for terrible back pain due to a herniated disc. She had great difficulty walking and had been all but confined to her sofa for six months. The strong narcotic painkillers her doctor had prescribed were no longer working. Her pain was continual.

Normally, Nola led an active life, but she now felt as if her life had been taken away from her. Being confined to her living room was not easy. She was on a waiting list for surgery. She did not like the idea of having the operation but felt it was her only option at this point.

During her first treatment she commented on how relaxed the CranioSacral Therapy made her feel. She giggled a bit and said that whatever I was doing felt like it did when her grandson drove his little cars around on her tummy. Her body's fascia and other soft tissues were releasing tension and realigning themselves. After this session, Nola reported being pain-free for two to three hours.

The second treatment, one week later, was much like the first. The difference was that during the latter part of the session, it felt as if gentle traction on the dural tube was causing a vacuum or suction effect within the tube; in turn this caused it to draw in toward its own center. Nola left the session feeling no pain and hoped that it would last longer this time.

A week later, when she arrived for her third treatment, she was ecstatic. She was completely pain-free and had given up all her pain medication. She said her doctor was surprised and impressed. He found it hard to believe that she no longer needed the pills he had been prescribing for so long. She reported being somewhat shaky and weepy but thought it was due to withdrawal from the drugs she had been taking for several months.

During the third treatment, as I followed Nola's bodily cues, I was led to do only a small amount of work regarding her back.

Most of the session seemed to be focused on what felt like cleaning out old issues or old material.

When I saw Nola a week later, she informed me that her whole life was changing. She had begun to clean out every nook and cranny of her house and was getting rid of all the hobby paraphernalia she had collected over many years. This was a very large amount, since she had owned a hobby store at one time. She then told me that as a young girl she had worked with horses and hoped to get back into it, probably in a volunteer capacity.

When Nola arrived the next week, she greeted me with the words, "You will never believe what happened!" (This is a phrase you get used to hearing when you practice CST.) The surgeon had reviewed her case, and the surgery had been canceled; he said there was no need for it.

In addition, a commercial building Nola and her husband had been trying to sell for some time finally sold. The purchasers were looking for acreage to house their four horses and would need someone to help look after them. The job went to Nola.

Nola continued in her weekly treatments for another month. After that she could not come as often because her horseback riding lessons were scheduled at the same time. She still pops in occasionally for a CranioSacral Therapy tune-up. It is several months now since she first came to see me. She is still pain-free, active, happy, and riding horses.

Iris Otterson, CST
Courtenay, British Columbia, Canada
CranioSacral Therapy Practitioner since 1998

Healing the Dance

Preparing to make a left turn, I looked in my side-view mirror but saw nothing in particular. (The fact that the mirror wasn't working correctly may have had something to do with it.) As soon as I turned, something hit the back of the car, and the left side of my head hit the car door. It hurt, but I found myself unable to tell people when they asked me if I was okay. Within a few minutes I regained my speaking ability. After talking to police and the driver of the other car, I drove home.

I took the next day off, thinking that the pain would go away. Instead, it took almost two years to recover from the constant pain, tinnitus, and migraines that the seemingly minor accident had started. I didn't work at all for six months after the accident, and worked only part-time for another six months after that.

As a physical therapist and massage therapist, I knew about CranioSacral Therapy (CST) and started to get treatment right away.

It is now thirteen years later, and I still receive CST to help with the headaches and back pain. I have a full life, filled with family, rewarding work, dance, and lots of play time with our daughter and five pets. Last year I even took my family to Florida, where I had three sessions with Dr. John [Upledger] himself.

The interesting thing was that my sessions with Dr. John were nothing like those with any other CranioSacral Therapist. Dr. John told me that he teaches therapists to use five grams of pressure, but with my body he used more, because he felt my membranes were so thick and, well, stubborn.

What happens during a CranioSacral Therapy session is that I suddenly feel understood. Medical doctors never diagnosed anything wrong with me. In fact, my disability insurance was denied because the doctors who examined me (and never touched me, by the way) said there was nothing wrong other than my complaining.

When Dr. John held my head and worked with it, it felt like he was stretching a muscle that had been held in a brace for twelve years. I could feel the stickiness in the motion in my head. I could feel the direction of the pulling, how it changed the alignment of my neck, my spine, my pelvis, my legs. When he held my left knee, it rotated my pelvis, and I finally felt comfort.

Then Dr. John unwound my spine by finding and loosening that place in my stomach where a knot of old and hardened tears had grown. It was at that point I remembered the shoes that a doctor had told my parents I needed to wear to prevent my feet from turning in. They were attached by a bar. I wore them at night when I was around four years old. I know it wasn't for long, because my mother and father agreed that I just cried too much when I wore them, and they gave up trying to fix me that way. Instead, my mom signed me up for ballet lessons. I'm not sure that was the best answer for my turning-in problem, though, because it altered my pelvis when I tried to turn out. Ironically, I became a dancer and a physical therapist, exploring and dancing my way through life despite tragedies and interruptions to living.

When Dr. John held my legs in this twisting, unwinding way, it was the opposite of everything I had tried not to do since I was four. It was like unraveling an old twisted-up sheet, the crevices filled with the dust of pain and tears, strains and sprains, memories of running and falling, toe shoes and rehearsals, New York City and competition, fat and skinny, abuse and abandonment, hope and renewal, and forgiveness.

Though we often start out thinking that what we're feeling is a purely physical thing, this work becomes emotional at the same time. With my background I understand what is happening; it is healing in motion. We are not two-dimensional beings, where a pain at this spot in our head is randomly connected to a spot in our necks. We are not three-dimensional beings, either, sculpted like clay and left to be looked at like a statue. We are four-dimensional (or more) beings, with motion and its kinetic effects coursing through every cell. Even in our quietest moments, there is pulse, rhythm, breath, and flow influencing every structure in our bodies.

Whatever this healing unfolds, because it includes motion in its definition, it recreates and catalyzes the release of all the sensations of the pain experience.

May Kesler, MS, PT
Washington, DC
CranioSacral Therapy Practitioner since 1995

Lilly's List

✿ Lilly is a woman in her seventies who works at the laundromat I use. Over the years we have struck up a friendship. Each time I took a healthcare class, I would tell her about it, and she would let me do a few small procedures on her.

Lilly had undergone several operations on her feet. As a result, she used a cane and tended to waddle when she walked in order to keep her balance. One could see from the look on her face that she was in pain.

After taking my first CranioSacral Therapy class, I approached Lilly about letting me do some work on her. She decided to give me a try because I had previously helped her arm feel better.

Immediately after I applied the 10-Step Protocol on her, she said that her hip felt better. The next time she went to work, her customers all commented on how her face just "glowed." They wanted to know what she had done. When I saw her, I was amazed. Her face really did have a glow about it.

After her third session, I asked Lilly to write down all the ways she had benefited from the CranioSacral Therapy so far. Here is what she wrote:

1. I don't bite the side of my mouth anymore.
2. My body feels back in line.
3. My sinuses don't bother me much.
4. I don't have headaches like before.
5. I walk straighter. [She doesn't waddle as much.]
6. I have more energy.
7. My ears don't bother me much anymore.
8. The arthritis in my shoulders doesn't hurt or ache as much.
9. I am more relaxed, so I sleep better.
10. I am able to breathe better.
11. I feel better about myself.

Gloria Andrews, kinesiologist
Newaygo, Michigan
CranioSacral Therapy Practitioner since 2002

The Case of the Missing Cerebellum

❁ When I first met Diana★ she had constant headaches, accompanied by migraines three to four times a week. She used medications as well as nerve pain for the migraines, but these only dulled the pain a little. Her headaches were so severe that she was forced to lie in a darkened room for several hours whenever they hit. Diana had three small children and was concerned for their safety. She also felt that she was not able to spend the time she wanted with them.

An MRI revealed that Diana was missing her right cerebellum, and the area that normally housed it had filled with fluid. The neurologist who referred her to me suggested that she may have had a stroke just before or after birth, which affected the cerebellum.

Although Diana's left cerebellum appeared to have taken over most of the functions that would have been done by the right side, she had always been clumsy in sports and had not walked until she was nineteen months old. (Her siblings had all begun to walk before they were a year old.) Diana had not been aware of this damage to her brain until her headaches sent her to the neurologist.

Treatment consisted of the 10-Step Protocol. When I began to mobilize the temporal bones, Diana remarked, "That really feels good." As the temporal bones were decompressed, her eyes flew open and she exclaimed, "Where did my headache go?!"

Diana left the office pain-free for the first time in several months. Her pain did not return for several hours. After her next treatment, her headache left for a day. Each treatment extended her headache-free time, and she also did not have any migraines for three weeks. At this point I discharged Diana, but she continued to take the migraine medicine "just in case."

Diana called a few weeks later to tell me that she was pregnant

---

★Name changed to protect client confidentiality

again and would not be able to continue taking her medication. She was afraid to stop without resuming therapy, so she returned for two more visits. The headaches did not come back.

More than a year later, Diana came in to have me work on the adhesions that formed after her C-section. She was happy to inform me that her headaches still had not returned.

Peggy Fye, OTR
Kansas City, Kansas
CranioSacral Therapy Practitioner since 1997

Riding the Waves to Healing

✿ I recently experienced my second bioaquatic session of CranioSacral Therapy. Going into it, I wasn't really suffering from any horrible pain, but I occasionally had sacral issues that flared up.

I had long suspected that a childhood injury in which I shattered my foot was causing some of the pain, as it was a "jamming" type of injury. I also had been involved in a very minor car accident about twelve years prior. The impact occurred on the driver's side at a very slow rate of speed. As the passenger, I got banged around a bit but nothing serious.

During this second bioaquatic session I had decided that I really wanted to talk to my body and explore these issues in order to rid myself of them. It was a beautiful day on Siesta Key Beach in Sarasota, and the water was crystal clear. I was the last session of the day. The surf was picking up a bit due to boating traffic nearby. The session started, and I began having a "discussion" with myself, saying it was okay to release whatever came up, but I would like to take a look at the sacral issues that were going on, if possible.

Within a few minutes I was in what my group called a "trance," as the waves kept going over my face and head. Somehow I never took in any saltwater.

During the thirty minutes of treatment, I stretched out and shrank into a fetal position a couple of times. I even rolled over in the water twice. At one point I could actually feel my sacrum starting to tingle—then I was hit with a remembrance of the car accident. The tingling stopped and I stretched out again. The tightness I had not even realized I was living with had totally dissipated.

I then experienced a variety of aches and even a burning sensation in my left foot and ankle (the one I broke years before). When members of my group tried to hold my ankle, I pulled that foot away, even though they were using only five grams of pressure. Then what came to me was a remembrance of a sledding accident. The next thing I knew, the pain was gone.

While I was completely conscious of what was going on, I felt that my body was determining what was going to happen, even to the point of regulating my breathing so that I didn't breathe as the waves crashed over my face. It was really an enlightening, beautiful experience as my body started learning to adapt to these new positions.

The session ended and I came back to the group of relative strangers who had supported my journey. I could actually feel my craniosacral rhythm come back on.

I have been pain-free in both my sacrum and left ankle for almost a month now. Even those close to me have remarked on the change in posture.

Thank you, Dr. Upledger, for this experience.

Michele Mathiesen, LMT, NMT
Sarasota, Florida
CranioSacral Therapy Practitioner since 2003

Do You Hear What I Hear?

✿ Judy* came to me for CranioSacral Therapy because she had heard that it helped with asthma problems. During my intake at our first meeting, I found that, along with the asthma, she also had hearing and other health problems.

I started working with Judy in the summer, and the CST helped tremendously with her asthma. Her doctor was amazed at her progress. She went from being on five different medications to taking them only as needed. We kept going into the fall and winter with the same results.

Around this time Judy's doctor suggested surgery on the bones of the ear to correct her hearing problem. She wanted to wait until after the holidays, however. In December she began to notice that she had to turn down her hearing aids because she seemed to hear better that way.

Then a remarkable thing happened.

A week before Christmas, Judy was downstairs in the kitchen, and her husband was upstairs in the living room. She yelled at him to get out of the candy jar. He asked how she knew he had taken some candy, and she told him that she heard him get into the jar. He then proceeded to tell her that she needed to instruct me to stop working on her ears, because he couldn't get away with getting into the candy jar anymore without her knowing.

Judy still has to wear the hearing aids, but she now has better hearing than ever before.

Pam Thurlow, LMT
Sanford, Maine
CranioSacral Therapy Practitioner since 1998

---

*Name changed to protect client confidentiality

Pat's Problem

❀ I have been doing alternative health therapy since 1998. I do a combination of things, such as health kinesiology, aromatherapy, brain gym, isometric muscle balancing, and CranioSacral Therapy.

In September 2003 I received a call from a man requesting an appointment. In his fifties, Pat* was a big, solid man of about three hundred sixty pounds.

The previous December Pat had gone out to his garage to untie his dog. When he bent over he lost his balance, fell on his forehead, and was instantly paralyzed. His arms drew up to his chest, his hands curled under, and he could not move his legs or anything.

At the hospital the paralysis left after about four or five hours, but his legs and arms were left feeling like they were asleep, with a numb/tingly feeling. He lost about eighty percent of the strength in his arms. For the next eight months, doctors ran a battery of tests to determine the reason for this, but nothing showed up. He was desperate. When he came to see me he walked like Frankenstein—very stiff-legged, not sure where his legs were.

I asked him if he had broken any bones. He said that X-rays indicated he had not. I then asked if the doctors knew the reason for his brief paralysis. They had told Pat that it was caused by the dural tube swelling. When the swelling went down, the paralysis left, but his legs and arms remained in this numb/tingly state.

I did some muscle testing, followed by the 10-Step Protocol. I found eight restrictions in the dural tube and was able to remove four.

After I finished, I told him if he felt even ten percent better, he should be encouraged. A profound amount of work had been accomplished. I asked him to come back in another two weeks, but

*Name changed to protect client confidentiality

he wanted to wait before he made another appointment. I don't think he believed I had done very much, and it did appear that way.

One week later Pat called for another appointment, saying that he was feeling at least eighty percent better. When he arrived at the office, I went out to meet him. Getting out of the truck he looked like he was barely touching the ground! I had to laugh out loud, because it brought such joy to my heart.

I did another 10-Step Protocol on Pat and removed two more restrictions. I told him to come back again one more time to finish up the work, but he did not keep his appointment.

Some time later, one of my clients said to me, "Do you remember Pat, who you worked on last year?"

I said, "How could I forget? I have always wondered what happened with him."

She said, "He told my granddaughter, 'You tell your grandmother thank you for telling me about Gloria.'" So Pat must be feeling okay.

Gloria Andrews, kinesiologist
Newaygo, Michigan
CranioSacral Therapy Practitioner since 2002

Menses Begin Again

❀ Through the course of more than five years traveling the globe, absorbing all kinds of different healing techniques and medicinal applications, and ten years of practicing holistic natural health, I encountered CranioSacral Therapy (CST) on a number of occasions.

A close friend who was a CST practitioner gave my family immeasurable comfort during three particularly traumatic years. With the use of CST primarily, my mother was comforted as she labored with lung cancer. Then my sister's firstborn was transformed at the age of only three months from a thoroughly unbalanced and unhappy screamer into a calm, responsive, and adorable bundle.

After a fairly challenging time in my own life, in which I suffered a brain hemorrhage for which I had to undergo brain surgery and months of recuperation, I was finally back on my feet and ready to tackle life again. To my joy, a long-awaited opportunity to study CranioSacral Therapy finally presented itself in Cape Town, my present home. I enrolled immediately and spent a hugely fascinating and enjoyable three days learning the technique.

If I had needed any further proof of the power of CST, or persuasion that it was meant for me, I was shown just that on our second day. I was lying down whilst my partner for the session was running through the 10-Step Protocol. She said she felt something was stuck down towards my lower abdomen on my left side. I was very curious since, to my knowledge, I had no problems whatsoever in that area of my body.

That evening, almost as soon as I arrived home, I began to feel a series of short but fairly sharp jabs of intermittent pain exactly where she had mentioned. Within twenty-four hours my menstrual cycle kicked in for the first time since my brain operation!

Amanda Whittle, ITEC
Wynberg, Cape Town, South Africa
CranioSacral Therapy Practitioner since 2003

My Dad's Heart

❀ Leading the family as we knelt in prayer, I felt a four-inch band of energy constrict around Dad's chest. Unaware of any physical problems, I urged Dad to mend any hurt feelings he may have felt or caused.

Two weeks later, Dad was in the hospital amidst a flurry of activity. Mom watched through the glass as doctors and nurses flew past her to apply electrical paddles to his chest. Though they had saved him to this point, tests showed that he had constrictive pericarditis. The heart's outer membrane had become a hardened, calcified shell, choking the inner muscle and its function in a progressive death grip. Surgical removal was necessary for survival.

My brother John and I flew in from the East and West coasts. We were in the waiting room with my mother and great-aunt when the doctor came and reported a successful surgery. Though he would have a difficult recovery ahead of him, Dad's situation was improved.

John spent virtually every day for three months in the hospital. I traveled back and forth between the hospital in Idaho and my home and job in California. We went together to the hospital library to read about Dad's diagnosis and surgery. We discovered that the expected recovery rate was a dismal fifty percent. We knew Dad would want us to fight for him.

For the next weeks, Dad was in and out of a mostly drug-induced coma. He had a few lucid moments to spend with us. On one of these occasions, he turned to me and remarked that the doctors knew all about surgeries and taking care of bodies, but that I had a gift of healing from God. He said he couldn't recover without my help. He got my promise that I would do whatever I could. The best I could do as a physical therapist was range of motion to keep his arms and legs flexible. Then there was CranioSacral Therapy.

The road to recovery was extremely difficult. There were times when twelve bags of IV fluids would be hanging at once. Twice they pumped him with heavy loads of fluid to get his circulation going, and then drained off sixty pounds of fluid within the next day. There were drugs to stabilize body functions and drugs to counteract the side effects of drugs. Our extended time in the coronary care unit was like science fiction—only it was real.

We asked hospital staff about Dad's progress on any given day, because we couldn't tell. He was comatose in appearance, and only they could unlock all the technology on the screens to read us his progress. We were fortunate to have a competent hospital team, yet we wondered if we would ever have our dad back fully alive, thinking and speaking normally with us again. It was a comfort to know that his initial craniosacral rhythm following surgery was good and strong. It made for a better survival outcome.

I remembered Dad's words about my helping him to heal. The nurses were very supportive and allowed me to work with him. When I was exhausted, Mom would put her hands on my shoulders and think good energy thoughts to keep it going. He was often so covered with various tubes and wires that I could only put my hands at his feet and do CranioSacral still points. I noted that every time he was put on the breathing machine, his craniosacral rhythm weakened, as if the machine were taking over everything. After he would come off, I "jump-started" his system again.

We used what skills and alternative healing methods we could. We brought in a green light for healing. We prayed. I had the opportunity to feel Dad's craniosacral rhythm strengthen directly, while John gave a blessing for rebuking an infection. Mom consulted our naturopath and persuaded the doctors to allow nutritional supplements to be pulverized and fed through the nasal-gastric feeding tube twice a day. She also had music and an essential oil diffuser brought in. We were Dad's healing team. I was surprised that the hospital staff was so indulgent with us.

There was a period of three days when Dad's blood pressure was dangerously low. We were not even to bump his bed, or he could die.

The time came for me to leave. Remembering Dad's words to me, I gave him a complete CST treatment the night before I left. I wedged myself between the headboard and the wall. I felt my energy meld with his while I worked on him for about an hour. I kept my eyes on the blood pressure monitor, hoping I wouldn't kill him with my efforts. Finally, his pressure began to go down and we left his room, hoping for the best.

I woke from a deep sleep at three-thirty the next morning. I felt the emotions of my dad's spirit coming back into a very broken body. It was terrifying. It was as though I was sharing a near-death experience with him. My shuttle left at six a.m. I wondered throughout the day how he was and if we had worked too hard to keep him with us.

I called that evening when I arrived home. Dad had gained consciousness that very day. He was talking and being himself.

Today, Dad is home. Although he doesn't remember specifics about his time in the hospital, he has had some terrifying feelings that he couldn't quite bring to the surface. As I described to him my early-morning experience of the spirit reuniting with body, it rang true to him. He has taken consolation from this story.

Dad has exceeded all expectations. He again is active in golfing and enjoys his grandchildren. We have been given a gift of his extended life to warm our own hearts.

Christine Perkins, PT
Turlock, California
CranioSacral Therapy Practitioner since 1999

CST Brings New View of Healthcare

As a practicing physical therapist for twenty-eight years, I have been taught to administer specific treatments that have been proven by quantifiable research and scientific study, and to look with skepticism on treatments that are verifiable only through clinical success stories. Therefore, it was with some wariness that I approached the study of CranioSacral Therapy (CST).

I am a newcomer to the field, having been introduced to CST while in massage school four years ago. My interest increased after I took CranioSacral Therapy, level one, and discovered the scientific rationale behind the treatments. Since then I have enthusiastically embraced CranioSacral Therapy and eagerly sought ways to promote its use.

Lecturing on CST one day before a business group to which I belong, I was approached by a member who suggested that her friend, Mrs. W,★ might be a good candidate.

Mrs. W was a forty-five-year-old nurse with a three-year history of unrelenting headaches and associated nausea. She had undergone microvascular nerve decompression as a treatment for trigeminal neuralgia. Recurring symptoms necessitated three more decompressions after that. Mrs. W developed inflammation in response to titanium mesh used during surgery and was treated with steroids. Then, a spinal tap revealed leakage of cerebrospinal fluid, an occurrence that ultimately required three shunts and six shunt revisions.

Mrs. W continued to experience severe headaches (level ten on a zero-to-ten scale) and nausea. This nausea resulted in progressive weight loss, since she did not feel like eating. She described the headaches as being "like a fist inside the head, pushing to get out." She was taking three separate prescription medications (including

---

★Name omitted to protect client confidentiality

narcotics) for headaches, none of which relieved the symptoms. She also reported continued trigeminal neuralgia symptoms.

Neither Mrs. W nor her husband, who was also an RN, had heard of CranioSacral Therapy, but they were receptive to any technique that might decrease her pain. I gave them a copy of Dr. Upledger's book, *CranioSacral Therapy: Touchstone for Natural Healing,* which they both read. Mrs. W's husband developed a particular interest in the concepts.

Initially I treated Mrs. W weekly for eight sessions. At the first session, I could only use one gram of pressure and no still points. Treatment consisted chiefly of diaphragm releases, which were adapted to Mrs. W's responses. She experienced both exacerbation and remission of symptoms. Immediately after that first session, she reported a decrease in headache pain from a level ten to level four.

At each successive treatment, Mrs. W experienced fewer symptom exacerbations and was able to tolerate longer sessions. She went from thirty minutes of complete relief from her headache after the first treatment to one week of complete relief from headache pain. Additionally, she was able to significantly reduce or eliminate the prescription medication.

At the fifth session, Mrs. W began experiencing emotional releases, but she was hesitant to allow them to release fully. Therefore, a counselor was called in on the sixth session to assist with the release process. (Mrs. W had previously described an especially traumatic emotional event in her past from which she thought she had recovered.)

Following the seventh session, Mrs. W's headache had resolved, and she was able to benefit from full CranioSacral sessions, including CV-4. Her nausea increased, however, and she continued to experience exacerbation and remission of the nausea.

By the tenth session, the nausea had decreased to level one, with the positive effects of therapy lasting two weeks. She was also able to completely discontinue the narcotics, and she could eat small amounts of food. After session eleven, Mrs. W reported no headache or nausea, and only minimal trigeminal symptoms.

At session twelve, Mrs. W's pain had changed to a different location and her nausea had increased in intensity. She began experiencing specific pains in the right upper quadrant of her abdomen. (She had previously reported that tests were negative for any organ problems.) At this point I felt that her symptoms might be better addressed by an advanced practitioner, and so I referred her to an advanced CranioSacral Therapist.

Through subsequent phone calls, Mrs. W related that three sessions with the advanced practitioner had allowed "good" emotional releases to occur, but were followed by intense exacerbation of the nausea. Therefore, she returned to her medical doctor for further evaluation and tests, specifically targeted at the gallbladder.

Although I and the other practitioner did not "cure" Mrs. W's symptoms, the CranioSacral techniques did facilitate the proper progression of healing for her body and allowed it to show us the probable source of the symptoms. By removing those symptoms that were masking the real problem, CST allowed the medical doctors to focus their attention on a specific area of complaint for which they could offer her a solution.

CranioSacral Therapy showed Mrs. W that her symptoms could be addressed by means other than medication and its related side effects. It showed her the strong and intimate connection between mind and body. And, above all, CST gave Mrs. W hope for a brighter future.

Mrs. W and I still keep in contact with each other. In fact, she has invited me to her daughter's wedding this summer. I thank both her and her husband for allowing me to be part of her healing process.

Alice Huss, PT, LMT, CPI
Albuquerque, New Mexico
CranioSacral Therapy Practitioner since 2003

A Change of Heart

❋ I have been practicing CranioSacral Therapy almost exclusively for more than two years at the community health center where I work with AIDS and HIV-positive individuals. In that time I have had several experiences that touched my heart and rekindled my spirit for this work.

One instance involved an HIV-positive man in his fifties who had taken a leave of absence from work for health reasons. He was scared, anxious, and depressed. He was unable to get himself out of bed and was surprised that he had made it in to see me that morning. He told me that he had been feeling lethargic, tired, unmotivated, and full of pain. He said, "I don't know what I'm going to do with my life; I want to go back to work." It was the first time in his adult life that he was not working and felt so ill.

When he came to see me, the man was expecting a regular massage. When I told him about CranioSacral Therapy and its benefits, he said that he'd like to try it.

After our first session, the pain-stricken client felt some improvement in levels of general body aches, and significant improvement in complaints of headaches. I encouraged him to come back in a week.

Upon coming for the second session, the man asked me, "What was it you called this work? I don't know what you did, but I felt really good this week." His pain had remained low for the rest of the week, and his spirits were starting to rise.

He continued to improve physically and emotionally. At our third session, he told me of all he had accomplished the previous week: working in his garden, fixing up the exterior of his house, and spending time with friends. He no longer looked or felt tired, nor did he have significant pain in his body.

Our fourth and final session was key for me. My client told me that he'd be returning to work the following week, something that he originally was hoping he could accomplish. Now his dilemma was no longer "How can I go back to work?" but "How do I sustain the joy of not working?"

In a matter of four sessions, my client had made a one-hundred-eighty-degree turn. He felt better about life and himself, and he no longer complained of body aches and pains.

Rich Kaminski Sol, LMT
Chicago, Illinois
CranioSacral Therapy Practitioner since 2002

Life or Afterlife?

❀ A man named John, age thirty-six and a competitive cyclist, came in for CranioSacral Therapy on March 31, 2004. He found CranioSacral Therapy through a TV program, and his wife rang me to arrange the visit.

Three years prior, John had broken his neck in a cycling accident and had gone into a coma that lasted three months. A big, strong man with a charismatic and gentle manner, he hadn't been able to work since. (He had been in sports sales.)

John had no memory of the accident. In fact, he didn't believe he had been in an accident at all. He actually thought he was dead and we were all in the afterlife.

After going through the rounds of medics, psychiatrists, and psychologists, John had given up. He had been off medication for four weeks at the time of his first visit with me.

I found him to be very intelligent and in good physical condition. He was also beyond persuasion. The psychiatrists termed his condition "derealization." The progress of our sessions was about establishing trust.

At John's fourth visit, he seemed to have lost all hope. He was still in the afterlife, but I knew he was ready to emerge from it. Working between the neck and heart area, testing the rhythms, we went piece by piece through the tissue back to the accident. It was a very deep and gentle session. By the end he had regained all of his memory.

After the session, we had a long conversation. John says he wants to go to University and rebuild his life slowly. I'll be seeing John again in two weeks' time.

Geraldine Nolan
Dublin, Ireland
CranioSacral Therapy Practitioner since 1999

A Surprising Result

❀ One never really knows the far-reaching effects that Cranio-Sacral Therapy will have on the lives of those who receive the work. It doesn't even have to be a lot of work to make a difference.

Here is a case in point I encountered as a CranioSacral Therapy instructor. On day three of class, the sphenobasilar compression/depression technique is taught during the afternoon. This technique is part of the 10-Step Protocol. It addresses a myriad of functions, including that of the pituitary gland, which is responsible for many metabolic activities.

The class format is fairly standard. A lecture is given, then a student in the class volunteers to be on the table so that the technique can be demonstrated by the instructor. The students then get to practice the technique on each other.

The next morning, before class began, the student who had been the demo person on the table the day before asked to speak to me privately. My curiosity was piqued, and of course I consented. She proceeded to tell me that she was married to an angel. My thought was, "That's nice." She went on to say that ever since her daughter was born twenty-one years before, she had not had a libido; her sex drive had been nonexistent. All that had changed the day before, however, after she had had her sphenoid worked on during the demonstration. To her amazement, and her husband's delight, that was no longer a problem!

We, as therapists, never know how our work is going to affect someone's quality of life. In all honesty, I could not recall what specific lesion patterns she exhibited the day before during the demonstration. It all goes back to Dr. John's [Upledger] teaching on how to listen to the body and treat what we find. The person on the table is our greatest teacher. As a therapist, I always ask that whatever happens be for the greater good. In this woman's case the outcome was a delightful surprise for her and her husband.

Shyamala Strack, OTR/L, CST-D
Atlanta, Georgia
CranioSacral Therapy Practitioner since 1991

Art, Yoga, and Life Enhanced

I met Rose, an artist and yoga and dance instructor, while living in Kauai, Hawaii. Rose suffered chronic neck pain and curvature of the spine. In addition, her nose was misaligned and her head tilted to the side.

One day during a yoga session she complained of shoulder and neck pain. I asked her if she was aware of CranioSacral Therapy. She said that she had been to a couple of sessions with another practitioner on the mainland some time ago. She asked me for an appointment.

I began our first session by working with the diaphragms and getting releases in the spine. Her spine was particularly responsive and realigned immediately. Another time we focused on bringing her nose back into alignment. We then worked together for two sessions to bring her head back into alignment.

At that point we agreed to meet and work in the ocean. With the assistance of the ocean and the dolphin energy, Rose's head and nose came back into alignment.

It has now been more than a year since the treatments. Rose reports that the alignment is still holding and she no longer has any pain. The healing seems complete. She also says that the experience greatly helped her yoga practice, and her art is developing in new ways.

It has been miraculous to observe Rose's release of past emotional traumas and to see how her artwork is now developing internationally, helping others in their healing process.

Carol Anne Munro
Calgary, Alberta, Canada
CranioSacral Therapy Practitioner since 1998

Heart to Heart

✿ My father had Alzheimer's. Throughout his illness I treated him with CranioSacral Therapy (CST) and massage—the prohibition against working on family members rendered moot.

In the beginning my mother would drive him twenty miles to my massage office. During these sessions my father talked about a lot of things. It was as if he wanted to share details about his life with someone who would remember for him.

As the disease progressed, his body became more sensitive to touch. It felt as if he were growing a thick undercoat to protect his soul. I shifted from what was helpful in the past to what was needed in the present—the blending skills that came from Dr. Upledger's teachings to listen to and respect the body's intelligence.

Eventually Father became so agitated in unfamiliar surroundings that travel in the car became dangerous. I continued working with him at his home, where the family had agreed to keep him for the duration of the illness.

CranioSacral Therapy was my special connection to my father. His body would respond by becoming still. His face would gain a peaceful yet tentative look, like he was on alert against any invasion of his private world. I could not help becoming excited when Father's craniosacral system related to my hands and let me go heart-to-heart with an otherwise lost part of him. Never once did he become agitated during a CST session. Sometimes he would even sleep afterwards, which was a huge relief to my mother.

Then came the fall, which resulted in a broken hip, surgery, and an infection. At that point we had to place him in a nursing home.

Now rigid and his eyes glazed over, Father's body began to shut down. During the last week of his life I took the role of night nurse, sleeping in a cot by his hospital bed since he would not be able to call for help if needed.

That first night I watched him writhe against the hourly insertion of a suction tube. I quickly learned to suction him myself, but I did it "cranially," meaning with utmost respect for his lips, his throat, and even the mucus. I talked to his body, promising cleanliness, which had always been important to this dying man.

"Daddy," I whispered, "I'm going to make you feel fresh! Lips, if you would like to open just a tiny bit, I will clean Mouth." It became extremely easy. In fact, he'd open his mouth as I approached!

The third night his lung congestion became more harrowing, and his body begged for relief. Through arcing I sensed a mass of energy in his chest. By this point I felt like I was losing my mind from lack of sleep, so a physician friend came to be with me as I attempted a silent somatic release.

The area around Father's bed felt cocoon-like and sacred. As I held my hands over his chest, I was open to anything that might aid his body's rite of passage. A bit of energy came up into my hands and soon was gliding out of his chest. Although I had no idea what was happening, I kept relaxed on the premise that his body knew what it needed and that I should just allow it to happen and not interfere.

The experience ended gracefully, and my Father moved into a more relaxed position. My doctor friend and I were stunned and exhilarated by this communication. There was no need to suction him again.

Five days later, my children arrived from California for what would be my last night shift at the hospital. They were at a loss when they saw the vestige of their grandfather, but the room was extremely peaceful since the energy extraction. The three of us laid our hands gently on his legs and spoke quietly about nothing special.

Then I felt him call to me. "What is it, Daddy?" I now had gotten so comfortable talking to my father's Inner Physician that I continued on in front of my children, who didn't seem at all surprised. There was something he needed.

I touched his face and words formed in my head. "Is Mary [my mother, his beloved wife] okay? Where is she? Will she be looked after?" The messages were as clear as any you would get while doing CST on a locked shoulder in a professional office setting.

"Mom is at home," I told him. "We'll all look after her." I could feel this absorb into him. "It's safe for you to go now if you want."

There was a definite pause, and motion in the room stopped. I looked into his eyes that had for months been glazed and dim, and he looked back at me with clear eyes, squeezed my hand, and let his Spirit drift out of his body.

I said to my children, "Grandpa is gone." They had witnessed a death done mindfully by a person with Alzheimer's disease. I knew there would be years to grieve, but I was filled with ecstasy right then. Here was a person who had perfectly communicated his last wishes through the cranial connection, despite being in the category of those supposedly least able to have intelligent awareness.

I have always been amazed at CranioSacral Therapy. With that has come a delicious delight at being allowed the opportunity to communicate with a holy aspect of another being. Before this experience, however, there was always a little embarrassment at the joy it brought me because I was being paid to do it. At my father's deathbed I opened myself to embarrassment and found comforting humility. It was not me that was special, but rather the work of John Upledger; I was another grateful practitioner.

Margery Summerfield, LMT
Wakefield, Michigan
CranioSacral Therapy Practitioner since 1993

The Power of Directed Intention

❀ It was late one evening, and I was on my last appointment. He was the father of my client Cara, whom I was seeing on a regular basis because of a car accident. She had scheduled her dad for a relaxing massage. The thing is, after you learn the possibilities of healing with CranioSacral Therapy (CST), you never do just a relaxing massage again. You are always looking to see how you can really help this person.

I had had a long day of back-to-back clients and was looking forward to going home to the family. I walked out of my room to greet Cara's dad. When he stood up, he was six feet five inches! I collapsed inside thinking, "Where am I going to muster the energy to work on this guy?" Just my luck, I have the tallest client of my career at the end of a long, hard day! I put on a broad smile, though, shook his hand and showed him into my room.

Immediately upon entering, he started reading my wall of diplomas, licenses, and certifications. He then pointed to my undergraduate diploma from State University of New York at Cortland back in 1972. It turned out he was the Chancellor of Education who signed the diploma! Now I really was motivated to give him a great massage.

His daughter mentioned to me that he had undergone recent surgery on his left shoulder and that it was really bothering him. I read his intake form and began. When I got to his left arm I tested his range of motion and found that it wasn't too bad. I did some directed energy holding techniques to help soften the fascia, which helped increase his range.

When I got to his right arm, though, it felt like a piece of wood. I had never felt anything like that before. He went on to tell me that he had injured it thirty-five years previously and had never followed through with his physical therapy. So his arm had been like that for all these years—stiff and with very limited range of motion.

Toward the end of the massage I asked Cara's dad if he would allow me to use some energy techniques on his shoulder. He agreed, so I proceeded to do the V-Spread technique that I learned in my second CranioSacral Therapy course. I directed the energy through what I now know to be a variety of specific acupuncture points or energy gateways. I then did directed energy, whole-hand, fascial-release techniques. As I worked, I could feel the hard tissue becoming alive under my hands. It was so amazing to me!

Even though I was so tired starting out, I completely lost track of time. When you're "inside" the healing experience, you're not finished until it's complete. You develop an intuitive sense as you do this work; you learn how to listen to the body. So when my client's body indicated it was finished for that session, he dressed, said goodbye and left.

As I was cleaning my room and putting new sheets on the massage table for the next day, I was startled by a loud, "Eileen, look!" There in the doorway was Cara's dad, showing me how high he was now able to lift his right arm. He reached all the way to the top of the door frame. We both stared in amazement. "I haven't been able to do that in thirty-five years," he said. "Thank you so much for giving me my arm back!"

This was my first real experiment using this wonderful work, CranioSacral Therapy. After that, I became a believer and knew that anything is possible!

Eileen Yocheved Hande, MA, LMT, CST
Boca Raton, Florida
CranioSacral Therapy Practitioner since 1993

A Single CST Session Preempts TMJ Surgery

❀ Two years ago, unbeknownst to me, my then twenty-eight-year-old daughter was battling temporomandibular joint syndrome (TMJ). She was at the point where she could eat only pureed foods with the use of a baby spoon and drink from a straw. Her physician had suggested surgery after all other Western medical modalities had been tried and failed to cure her painful, bothersome TMJ.

When she phoned to inform me of this, I told her to curtail surgery and come instead to my home, and I would perform CranioSacral Therapy (CST). She was very open to this.

When she arrived, I had the ambiance in my living room prepared with a few candles, soft lighting, and meditation music. I performed CST on her for about one and a half hours. She commented following the session that she felt as if her head and jaw were moving in all directions, although both had remained still throughout the session. She also stated that she felt a "gush of water" drain from her skull to her feet and saw numerous colors during the session.

Approximately fifteen minutes after the session, she started to have severe chills to the point of requiring two sweaters in an attempt to warm up. I informed her that this does happen occasionally. After about an hour, she left to go home.

My daughter has never been bothered by TMJ since that Cranio-Sacral Therapy session. She informed her physician of the CST work she received, and he was quite impressed.

I personally and professionally think this is fantastic. I am so grateful to have taken the training in CranioSacral Therapy so that I could give my daughter this remarkable gift and save her from going through with surgery.

Claudette L. Cyr, LPN
Sabattus, Maine
CranioSacral Therapy Practitioner since 2000

Alterations

✻ A vivacious young woman came to my treatment room one day. She complained that she was unable to take long car trips without stopping every forty-five minutes to get out, stretch, and walk. If she didn't, she would suffer severe hip and leg pain. In addition, her hip joints would pop when she climbed stairs, her left shoulder joint would grind with movement, and she had a lot of muscular tension and soreness.

The woman had been treated for scoliosis since she was a child. She had been forced to wear a body cast for this condition from the ages of ten to twelve. She was rarely comfortable in her body at any time.

About two years ago, her temporomandibular joint dislocated while she was yawning, and her jaw locked. This condition required arthroscopic surgery. She had experienced frequent pain in her head and neck ever since.

I evaluated this young lady and palpated a very pronounced scoliosis of the spine. The dural membrane felt restricted in many places in the spine and the cranium. Her left mandible was quite compressed into the temporomandibular joint, and the muscles in that area were very sore to even a light touch. This young lady had great vitality and very strong underlying good health, despite the obvious painful conditions she was experiencing.

She came to see me for CranioSacral Therapy (CST) once a week over four weeks. Her body changed with each visit. After her first session, she reported feeling more relaxed but said that some muscles felt sore after the treatment. After the next visit, her knee and hip popping was much improved, and she had less soreness when sitting for long periods. After the third visit, she said her jaw did not hurt and her hips felt more level when standing.

At the fourth visit, she said that she had recently been shopping for clothes. Prior to receiving CranioSacral Therapy, she had to have pants and skirts altered so that the hems would appear the same length. She was very surprised when she did not have to do this with her new clothes to accommodate a difference in leg length.

She also noticed that she could stand with her weight evenly balanced on both feet, and her hips were quite straight and level. She then told me she had a tattoo on her right hip that had moved since our last session; it was now lower and more to the side. She could not believe that her body had untwisted so much.

In addition, she said she had taken a car trip with her family and had been able to go the entire distance of two hours without having to stop and get out to stretch the way she normally did. This client's primary goal was to be able to take car trips with her family without discomfort. She improved quite rapidly with CST, achieving more relief than I expected.

The joint problem in her jaw recurred after one of our visits and lasted about a week. This pain cleared completely after the next treatment. Her chronic head and neck pain also stopped and did not recur. This young lady comes in occasionally for a CranioSacral Therapy tune-up. She has maintained the progress she made during her four weekly visits.

She returned a few months ago complaining of numbness in her right leg, which had always been her worst side. She said the problem started occurring after she bought a new car.

After our session, we went out to her car, and I adjusted the seat by adding a towel behind her back at the lumbar area. Making this adjustment moved her forward so that her hips and legs fit in the seat better. She called the next day to report that she had experienced no more problems with leg numbness. This client is very pleased with the alterations CranioSacral Therapy has made in her life.

Doris Weiner, RMT
Plano, Texas
CranioSacral Therapy Practitioner since 2000

Out of the Woods

❀ I attended my first CranioSacral Therapy class two years after I opened my massage therapy practice. A few months after that, my client Karen asked me to see her friend Jerry, who was "recovering from an illness." When I asked her what illness he was dealing with, she was vague. She said he had suffered a stroke and that few results had been gained from physical, occupational, water, and speech therapies. He was depressed, and she thought a massage might help him to relax and mellow out.

Upon meeting Jerry I learned that he had gone undiagnosed for two weeks while in the hospital. Doctors eventually surmised that he had contracted an infection from a tick or bug, which had infected his brain. (Jerry had worked for the Forestry Service and loved the outdoors.) He then had a stroke.

In his early seventies, Jerry was now largely confined to a wheelchair. He was unable to walk without being assisted by someone holding onto his gait belt. His arms were contracted up against his chest. His legs were unable to straighten completely. His whole body was racked with periodic spasms. And he was unable to speak more than two or three words at a time. He had been in this present condition for months with little or no improvement.

I talked with Jerry and explained what I would be doing. In place of massage, I opted to try and balance his energy system and ideally help him to relax somewhat.

While I put my hands at his feet, his body just radiated chaos. I was so afraid of Jerry having a violent response after seeing how his body periodically spasmed. His body had to be cushioned with large pillows, since he was unable to lie flat due to the contracted state of his arms, legs and back. I kept checking in with him to make sure he was okay with what was going on. I had a sense that his system was trying to "coordinate" itself. I also had a sense that he was nervous (no more than me!) and wanted to participate in his therapy but was unable to at the level he wanted. By the end of the session, he appeared more relaxed and looked like he wanted to sleep.

I worked on Jerry for an hour and then talked to him about allowing a therapist friend of mine to join me next time to assist with CranioSacral Therapy. Both Jerry and Karen agreed, even though neither one had heard of CranioSacral Therapy.

At the next visit we repeated what I had done the previous session, which was to get Jerry's system to relax through diaphragmatic holds as his body instructed us. Upon initial observation, I saw that his rhythm was not symmetrical. It was low amplitude, poor quality, and very chaotic. His breathing was shallow and his body occasionally spasmed. He also had rapid eye movement.

Jerry enjoyed the sessions. We continued to see him on a weekly and biweekly basis.

Then a CranioSacral Therapy study group learned about Jerry. They responded with excitement and wanted to help. On average we had four to six people working on Jerry simultaneously. He would go into full-body unwinds, with one person holding a limb, one holding his head, and another his chest or sacrum.

After a few sessions we noticed that Jerry was more alert and would follow our whispers with interest. His sense of humor began to return. As the sessions went on, Jerry began to speak more. Eventually he began to relate his bodily sensations during the sessions, along with his frustration at the lack of progress he experienced with other therapies. He was angry that he had lost his former lifestyle, and he did not have high hopes of ever returning to his former self. He did, however, want to improve as much as possible.

As Jerry began to feel his body responding to the sessions, he had trouble sitting still. He wanted to hurry things along by moving his limbs quickly when he felt a sense of renewed freedom in them. We encouraged his enthusiasm but gently reminded him to allow the process to happen.

The sessions went on for several months and Jerry steadily improved. His speech became easier to understand, and he was able to say whole sentences, make jokes, and give better feedback during his sessions. As his body slowly unwound and loosened, he began to believe he would get better.

Along with CranioSacral Therapy, Jerry continued to receive speech and water therapy. We watched as his arms were able to slowly move from their contracted position against his chest to lying down at his sides. His walk became more stable after a few months. His bowel function and appetite also improved.

During Jerry's next-to-last session we were amazed by the fruits of our work together. Upon Jerry's arrival, I had the privilege of seeing him emerge unassisted from the passenger side of the vehicle. I called out to everyone, "Look who's here!" As everyone turned, Jerry walked into the office on his own with a big smile on his face. There were many tears of joy flowing that morning.

After a few months I spoke to Karen on the phone. I discovered that they were going their separate ways and that Jerry would be moving away. Though I never saw Jerry again, I know that he had regained most of his mobility, cognitive functioning, speech and, more importantly, his dignity.

Lucy Franqui Gustitis, NCTMB
Kalispell, Montana
CranioSacral Therapy Practitioner since 2000

Sacred Passing

✿ There are many wonderful stories that speak to the positive impacts of CranioSacral Therapy (CST) in people's lives. Death is also a part of living, and I would like to share a story about how I think one special moment of still point intention may have helped my mother make an important transition in her process of dying.

My eighty-year-old mother had been in an intensive care unit for ten days, rushed from a nursing home to the hospital with breathing problems. This was the first time we had been faced with the question of resuscitation.

Historically, her lungs had not been the problem. My mother was diagnosed with Parkinson's disease about sixteen years earlier, and we had all observed a gradual decline in her abilities, though her health had remained stable. After four months of living in a nursing home, however, she showed a sudden downturn in her health: poor eating, weight loss, and probable anoxic episodes.

Early in the ICU admission, I had asked my mother what she wished with regard to further medical intervention. She was clear in her response that if her heart stopped, she did not wish to have the doctors start it beating again. I was grateful that she had been given a window of grace, a time during which my brother and father could come to terms with their own feelings about letting my mother go.

After much soul-searching, decisions were made to continue comfort measures but to withhold any further heroic cardiac or respiratory interventions.

On the night that my mother died, I arrived at the hospital around five p.m. She looked like she was sleeping, an oxygen mask covering her nose and mouth. Although she had been interacting with my brother the night before, my mother had been in this "deep sleep" state all day, unresponsive to any kind of stimuli, according to an ICU nurse.

Now that decisions about heroic measures had been made, the ICU staff began preparations to transfer my mother to another floor, which offered an intermediate level of care. While the oxygen mask, feeding tube, and intravenous line for medications all remained, the monitors indicating her vital signs were turned off. The silence became stunning and eerie to us. For our own comfort levels, we asked to have the monitors sent with my mother to the next unit.

When she was settled in, my father, brother, sister-in-law, and I gathered with her, recognizing that her end was probably near, although we did not have a sense of timing. My dad sat at my mother's left side, holding her hand. I sat at her right side, my hand slightly on her forearm, and periodically I was aware of her craniosacral rhythm.

It was close to ten p.m., and I cannot say exactly what prompted me to think about inducing a still point in my mother. In my early CranioSacral Therapy classes I had been taught that one would generally induce a still point by holding the craniosacral rhythm on the inward motion. In my recollection, it had been stated that to hold it on the outward motion might have an agitating effect, which was usually undesirable unless perhaps the person was in a coma.

It suddenly occurred to me that because my mother was in a comatose-type state, this form of still point might have some benefit. I wondered if it might stir her consciousness or perk her up a little.

Without further thought or expectation about what might happen, I followed the rhythm in her forearm through a few cycles and then quietly focused on holding the rhythm still as it moved toward the outward excursion. Immediately, we all heard a shift in the beeping of the heart-rate monitor. My mother's heart rate had dropped from a consistent one hundred ten beats per minute to eighty-eight, and it stayed there.

My brother, suspecting an impact from a dose of Lasix administered about ten minutes before, went to get the nurse. Upon seeing the situation, she suggested that Mother's heart was not working so hard now.

Privately, I was aware that the dramatic drop had coincided instantaneously with the still point, but this didn't seem to be the right place or time to try and explain. From a previous conversation with a nurse at the nursing home, I knew that my mother's heart rate had a standard of being high. Although I did not know what had just happened within her, I felt that a significant shift had taken place. I was not aware of any changes in her breathing pattern or in her facial expression. It was the heart-rate monitor that gave me feedback about a less obvious, but perhaps important, transition.

Within the next twenty-five minutes or so, my mother's heart stopped. At various intervals, I turned on the monitor. Dad and I noticed that her heart rate had lowered into the sixties and then the thirties.

Her final breaths were slow and drawn out with long pauses in between. The visible pulse in her neck became diminished. The final reading on the monitor showed a flicker of graph movement before it stopped.

I continued to monitor my mother's craniosacral rhythm. It still felt strong and steady. After about half an hour, I felt it come to a slow stop and then fade. I shared this with my family. By then everyone had felt a shift in the room, and we collectively knew that it was okay to leave. I don't think any of us could have left the room prior to the sense of completion, which seemed to occur at the same time as the stopping of my mother's craniosacral rhythm.

Three and a half years have since passed. It is my sense that the still point helped my mother in her process of letting go and moving on. It is my honor to have been witness to this sacred moment.

Pat Joyce, OTR/L
Amherst, Massachusetts
CranioSacral Therapy Practitioner since 1991

To Feel Again

As an occupational therapist for a home-health company, I was visiting a client who was suffering symptoms from a stroke. Her personal care assistant asked if she could watch me as I performed a CranioSacral Therapy session. Both the client and I agreed. Once finished, my client had more range of motion and balance as we practiced transfers.

The assistant began asking a number of questions about the treatment procedures, so I told her that it was easier to let her experience it than try to explain it to her. She consented and lay down on the couch. I did a thoracic outlet diaphragm release, a decompression of the occiput from the atlas, and one still point.

She lay very still for a moment or two then opened her eyes and began to cry profusely. I rested a hand on her shoulder and just waited.

When she finished crying she began to tell me that she had been unable to feel any sensation at all from her head down to her feet for over two years. She had been to a number of doctors and had finally given up hope of ever feeling her body again. She told me that when I took my hands away from her head, her whole body went cold and she could feel every one of her body parts.

She threw her arms around my neck and thanked me. For a moment all three of us shared her tears of joy.

We never know what is about to happen when someone asks us to step into their world with our touch.

Bob Munster, OT
Monroe, Maine
CranioSacral Therapy Practitioner since 1995

Try a Little Tenderness

✿ You know the saying "I feel like I've been hit by a bus!"? Well, my client *was* hit two years ago. It was one of those bizarre incidents of being in the absolutely wrong place at the wrong time.

Robyn, a petite, dark-haired young woman, was innocently crossing a busy street in the city center of Sydney, Australia, when a bus surged through the red light and struck her on the shoulder. She fell, striking her head on the pavement, which put her into a coma for three days.

Diagnosed with a bleed in the brain, Robyn sustained injuries of a closed-head nature. A year later the neurologists could find no indication of brain damage. Robyn still reported symptoms of headaches, reduced concentration, pain in her left shoulder with restricted movement, depression, and sleep disturbances.

Unfortunately, as is often the case, Robyn now had to put more effort into proving to the insurance companies that she had problems in order to receive some compensation for her injuries. (This is why my work with clients often begins with enlisting their willingness and desire to want to get better. Otherwise, they may unconsciously be working to maintain the problem so that the insurance company will believe they suffered a disabling injury.)

Another CranioSacral Therapy practitioner who had given Robyn a few sessions referred her to me. She found that more Somato-Emotional Release work needed to be done, and she thought that I might be able to address this more fully with the client.

Robyn's symptoms were chronic pain in her neck, muscles and nerves, headaches, an inability to sleep, anxiety with post-traumatic stress, depression, and listlessness. She had been unable to work for the past two years due to the poor concentration, depression, and low energy. She had weakened eyesight and was unable to sit for long periods due to shoulder and back pain, particularly on the injured left side.

My work with clients is primarily CranioSacral Therapy combined with Positional Release, massage, and acupressure. My intention and support of the client is for the renewed integration of his or her body/mind. I find that this is made possible with Somato-Emotional Release, which is the added component of finding the root cause to the disharmony within the body.

Before Hippocrates, the practice of medicine was known as theurgic. Theurgic medicine saw health as a relationship to the spirit or the divine, and illness as a loss of that relationship. Essentially I see my job as being a co-facilitator and co-creator in the healing process to establish a body/mind re-education of a person's physical body as well as his or her emotional and spiritual well-being. My belief is that this supports, encourages, and creates an integration of body, mind, and spirit.

Robyn's body at first touch was tense and holding, her head and upper thoracic area vise-like. There was an overall compression of the cranial bones and rigidity in her shoulders through the intercostal rib cage. After a general listening, I began with a simple cranial vault hold. She described "feeling lots of tenderness as well as numbness." This sense of tenderness, which I felt in her tissues, led me to first blend my hands into her tissue, as if I were able to manually *become* tenderness. I suggested then that she allow her body to float into that feeling, as if it were a bath or an ocean. It was what her body described to me nonverbally, and this was my interpretation. Having a felt sense with the client invites me into a healing space, where I can become a supportive witness on a fluid level to the process going on inside her body.

In this first session we found a meeting place of gentle, resting tenderness. Robyn's body spontaneously released in a full myofascial arcing movement, from the falx cerebelli to her sacrum, in an undulation of full fascial release. Throughout this process, I spoke quietly to her nervous system, which was responding to Robyn's feelings of raw nerves that were in panic and darkness. I reassured the nervous system that it had indeed been through a rough time.

I told her tissues and nerves that we were there to guide them back into a more relaxed state. I let them know that they had done a very good job keeping Robyn healthy, alert, and alive, but now they (the nerves) just needed a rest.

During our second session, I again began with this attitude of tenderness. As I moved into her left side, into the intercostal tissues, I asked her what had been happening in her life just before the accident. Had there been any life changes or experiences? Robyn expressed that she had broken up with her boyfriend of two years just before the accident. She then said, "I believe this accident happened for a reason." We had begun the journey of healing.

At our next session a week later, other long-held emotions surfaced. By the end, we were able to break through the layers of pain and grief.

By our follow-up appointment, Robyn reported that she felt much better, was no longer depressed, was able to take full breaths, and was able to sleep six hours a night. She was reading Russian literature and enjoying playing with paints in the garden.

Robyn still has some work to do in her healing process, but she is no longer suffocated by her life or the past. The accident is no longer the cause of her problems, and insurance is not her worst nightmare. More importantly, Robyn has a far greater tenderness for herself and her outlook on life.

Rebecca M. Ridge, MA, LMT
Anoka, Minnesota
CranioSacral Therapy Practitioner since 1986

Happy Migraines

✿ I met Christine shortly before this story was written. She had come to me for help with debilitating migraine headaches. She had never heard of CranioSacral Therapy (CST) yet was completely willing to try it. She experienced incredible empowerment right from the first session. I was especially pleased that her need for medication dropped dramatically, giving her positive reinforcement that she was in charge.

My treatment approach has been to simply follow my hands and "talk to the body." This has included talking to her headaches, discovering their purpose, and eventually offering them a new job and new name to match. At this point, Christine has had about twelve hours of CranioSacral Therapy over five sessions. Here is her story in her own words.

"For the past twenty-four years I have been dealing with and fighting migraine headaches. I was given a number of explanations by doctors: That's just the way it is. It might be hereditary. You should avoid all the trigger foods. Blah, blah, blah.

"Having watched my mother suffer with migraines, my sister for the past ten years, and my dad on occasion, I was not looking forward to a future of migraines. Lucky family we are!

"My sister Sheri heard first of Cathie, and we both instantly wanted to go. I had been on a mission for quite a while to learn and seek out the absolute best health for myself by whatever means were available to me. The way it usually worked was I did the experimenting, researching, and trying, and then whatever approach I found worked best for me, my sister did the same. Needless to say, I went to Cathie first—not that I minded in the least.

"My first thoughts of what might happen were that she would give me some self-help techniques for dealing with my body's many problems. In November 1999 I was diagnosed with high blood pressure, then kidney stones, then hyperparathyroidism. I was a mess. January 2000 brought two thyroid surgeries. The first one failed. In the second one, they removed my left thyroid and thymus and scraped my chest cavity. Needless to say, I have not been the same since—not like I wanted to be, anyway.

"Even though I didn't know what to expect from CranioSacral Therapy, I was determined and sure that Cathie was going to be able to help me help myself. I can now say that I am thoroughly convinced of CST's capabilities and completely ecstatic with what she and I have done together.

"The first session was quite amazing. My body told Cathie to go to my left jaw and neck area, which is the trigger side for my migraines. Turns out there was quite a bit of leftover baggage I was hanging onto. I ground my teeth as a child and sometimes in my adult years. As a teenager I had braces, all four wisdom teeth surgically removed, and was rear-ended by a tow truck at seventeen.

"As I write this, I have not had one migraine in the last five months. I have had many migraines come around knocking to get in, but since seeing Cathie I have been successful at sending them away. On one occasion I turned to the left toward the sound/sensation, and when I faced forward I had a wild rush of pain in my left temple. I quickly said, "No way, you are not welcome here anymore," and there it went. I was quite dizzy, as the feeling was very overwhelming and powerful. It was such a rush.

"I have asked Cathie at least once, 'Where were you twenty-four years ago when I really needed you?' Her answer: 'Out having fun, riding my motorcycle.'

"For twenty-four years I may not have been open and ready for someone like Cathie, but I am so happy and grateful to have found her now.

"Cathie and I have since spoken to Migraine and kindly asked it to take all that extra, awesome energy and help my thyroid and metabolism to become stronger and healthier. That was just yes-terday, and I can already feel a huge difference. That's why I now say I have happy migraines. I can hardly wait to see what happens next!"

Cathie Grindler
Richmond, British Columbia, Canada
CranioSacral Therapy Practitioner since 2002

Mother/Infant Bonding Restored

❀ Mrs. Montgomery* delivered a healthy, five-pound, fourteen-ounce girl by cesarean section. By five weeks the baby was thriving at eight pounds, two ounces—Mrs. Montgomery, however, was not. She was miserable with sore, misshapen nipples from the baby's feeding. She saw a lactation consultant, who made a referral for CranioSacral Therapy (CST).

At the time of our first visit, Mrs. Montgomery was trying a variety of alternatives to the breast, including a cup, finger, syringe, Avent bottle, and Haberman feeder. My initial evaluation indicated a number of strengths in the situation, including a dedicated mother, a baby happy to go to the breast, and plenty of milk.

Armed with this information, I set about developing a lactation care plan that included teaching the mother how to position her baby at the breast for ultimate comfort and milk transfer, and how to use co-bathing for pleasure. I also encouraged her to just pump her milk for twenty-four to forty-eight hours and let her husband feed the baby while she rested in bed.

Also at this first visit, the mother received CST at her feet, thighs, and ilia, as well as a lumbosacral decompression, some pelvic diaphragm releases, and sacral traction. The baby received CST while she was lying on her mother's chest. In particular, I worked on her dural tube, achieving releases in the vomer bone and cranial base. Both mother and baby experienced multiple, deep still points and reached a state of deep relaxation together.

During the next eighteen days, Mrs. Montgomery and I spoke on the telephone three times. Despite a steady improvement in breastfeeding comfort, the mother was not thrilled or happy. This was odd, because women are usually delighted when breastfeeding is finally easier and more comfortable.

---

*Names changed to protect patient confidentiality

At a second session, I worked with the mother extensively, holding an intention of unconditional, positive regard while doing the therapy. The mother received additional CST, experiencing releases in her fascia and more still points. During the session she volunteered that there was more going on with her than just "this breast-feeding stuff."

Mrs. Montgomery spoke and wept about various issues regarding mothering. She doubted she could be a good mother. Her confidence was received with empathetic listening, validation of the difficulties she was suffering, praise for the hard work she had been doing so well, and a suggestion that she continue her work with her therapist, whom she had not seen since late in pregnancy.

Following this second CST session, Mrs. Montgomery was able to easily maintain her breastfeeding relationship. Without CST in this case, one wonders if breastfeeding would have continued, as mothers need to enjoy this bond to sustain it.

Shelly★ was referred to me for CranioSacral Therapy by a fellow lactation consultant after breast problems persisted following accidental premature weaning.

At the time of our first visit, Shelly's son was eight weeks old. She was still breastfeeding on demand, pumping, and using each breast several times during a breastfeeding session. We developed a care plan to deal with the oversupply and with the nipple vasospasm.

Moving to the baby, initial assessment revealed bilateral parietal/temporal overrides ("corners"). He didn't want anything in his mouth. He placed my finger at his left maxilla, and I did a direction of energy to the corner on that side. There was significant occipital-cranial base release and dural tube unwinding to the left.

Over the next week his latch improved, and he opened his mouth wider. Shelly's supply began to regulate for one baby. The best feeds were accomplished lying down in bed at night. The possibility of reflux in the baby was ruled out by the pediatrician.

When I saw Shelly and the baby a week later, the baby nursed seven times in two hours at my office. Shelly commented, "He usually never breastfeeds during the day!"

I did some more regional tissue releases of his head to the left and his sacrum to the right. His head "corners" had rounded. Shelly also benefited from a good cranial base release and multiple still points, one while the baby was nursing lying on her chest. Both were very deeply relaxed by the time they left. I told her that she would probably be able to nurse in any position now.

At the end of our relationship she said, "This was the first difficulty I have ever conquered in my life."

Nikki Lee, RN, MS, IBCLC
Elkins Park, Pennsylvania
CranioSacral Therapy Practitioner since 1997

Living Pain-Free

❀ Following my first CranioSacral Therapy class, I was very eager to get back to my shop in rural southside Virginia so I could share what I had learned with my customers.

After returning home, I was disappointed to find that people who came into my shop with pain and headaches looked at me with suspicion when I told them about my new methods. They would take advice about herbs, but it sometimes felt like an uphill battle to get them to try anything that was different from orthodox medical practices. Even when I offered treatments without charge, I got very few takers and no repeat customers. I was beginning to wonder if I was doing something wrong or if I would ever be able to use my newfound knowledge.

After several months, a teacher in her early forties came into my shop. She was in obvious pain and desperately looking for some type of help. She had recently had an MRI that revealed a bulging disc, bone spurs, arthritis, stenosis, sclerosis, and degenerative disc disease of the lower lumbar area. The medical community had only offered her one option: spinal surgery. Even then there was no guarantee that the pain would end.

Being a teacher of small children, she was no longer able to do her job. She could not sit at the low tables, dance with her kids, bend over to zip coats, or even tie a shoe. She was suffering from fatigue because sleep was almost impossible from the pain that shot through her body every time she moved in bed. She said that one of her greatest fears was catching a cold because she knew that even a simple sneeze or cough would send pain coursing through her body.

She had already tried various herbal and homeopathic remedies that helped a little, but none had provided anywhere near the relief she needed. The only option she could see was giving up the job she loved because it hurt too much to do even the simplest of tasks. She also explained that surgery was not an option because she lived with her mother who was in her eighties, and there would be no one to care for her during the recovery period.

As she told her story, my mind raced to the things I had learned during my classes. Could CranioSacral Therapy help her? I was almost too nervous to even hope. I quickly explained what I had learned about energy blockages and how you have to clear the blockage so the blood can flow to the area and healing begin. All the while I was waiting for her to just turn and walk away. To my surprise, she agreed to let me try to help her, and we immediately began our first session.

Initially, lying on the table was almost impossible, and she could not lower her legs at all. When I put my hands on her lower back and began treatment, I did not feel anything for a long time. Once again my old fears stirred in my mind. Then I began to feel the slightest pulse. Suddenly it was like a dam breaking loose, and the pulse started to come stronger. Finally the first session was over.

Hoping I had brought an immediate relief to her pain, I was so disappointed when she indicated that the pain was actually worse right after the treatment. She had a terrible time getting off the table, and I had to help her put her shoes back on. She left, promising to let me know how she was doing and whether she wanted to come back for another treatment.

In a few days I heard back. She indicated that while the pain had been worse right after the first treatment, within a few hours she noticed a relief from pain without having to take powerful painkillers. She was so excited to think that finally there was a possible nonsurgical answer to her back pain.

After that, we had biweekly then weekly sessions. The pain always seemed much worse right after I finished the treatment. I began to notice, though, that her legs were lowering slowly. Then came the day I noticed that she was lying flat on the treatment table. She also did not need assistance getting up or putting on her shoes anymore. Soon she was strong enough to begin exercising and stretching her back.

Now, less than a year later, she is back in her classroom teaching. She can touch her toes, climb stairs, and even run. She is once again sleeping at night and is pain-free ninety-eight percent of the time. She continues to exercise and take her anti-inflammatory herbs and is able to lead a normal, happy life.

Through her testimony, more people are now listening. They are willing to try CranioSacral Therapy for themselves and recommend it to those they know. I have seen many people find relief from headaches and pain thanks to my newfound skills. For this I am eternally grateful.

Karl Simon, ND, MH
Clarksville, Virginia
CranioSacral Therapy Practitioner since 2003

Being Lost

✿ Looking back at some of my most memorable life experiences, I have come to realize that I often enjoyed being lost. There was a thrill to allowing myself lost time in a new city or country. It was a free-form way to explore, to open myself to people, surroundings, and pastimes. Being lost was like a trip without a tour guide, going with the flow of whatever I encountered. I never got into serious trouble, and I could always somehow find my way home. Being lost was play.

There was another kind of lost, however, that took me quite a while to experience in such a positive light. This was the lostness I felt from the chronic pain and inflammation of rheumatoid arthritis.

In my early forties I began experiencing gradually worsening musculoskeletal pain associated with running, swimming, and my work as a pediatric physical therapist. As the chronic inflammation reached a fairly high level, I sought answers and additional help.

I started by taking a Myofascial Release course. This was new territory for me, combining very deep, Swedish massage-type bodywork with the gentle craniosacral invitation to allow the fluids to flow. It unleashed an inflammatory response in my body that left me helpless with joint and ear pain, joint swelling, and immobility.

In this instance of being lost, there was no helpful gas station attendant, hastily purchased map, or readily apparent inner sense of knowing I could turn to to get me home. It was the early 1990s, and the medical breakthroughs we now have did not yet exist.

With the help of anti-inflammatory and immunosuppressant medications, I avoided major permanent joint damage. I was able to struggle to continue with work, a life with my family, and the pursuit of some kind of inner compass. This was a prolonged period of feeling deeply lost in pain, fatigue, anger, and distrust.

All was not lost, though. My experience with Myofascial Release left me with the knowledge that bodywork is terribly powerful. My inner knowing told me that if this bodywork was done right, I was going to be able to find my way home.

I took John Upledger's CranioSacral Therapy (CST) classes as quickly as I could and busily began to practice. I was amazed at the kinds of changes I felt under my hands and the kinds of results those receiving CST were experiencing. I was thankful that I had found a new, gentle way to interact as a therapist that was both effective and did not overly tax my arthritis-diminished work capacities.

I have to admit, though, that I did not get a lot of the Cranio-Sacral work done on myself in those days. I did not listen to my inner knowing. It was not until I took Advanced CranioSacral Therapy that my inner knowing received a rude awakening. My lack of receiving was a big source of my being lost.

Receiving CranioSacral Therapy on a regular basis over the past five to six years has made being lost fun again. The gentle following and encouragement of my therapists has allowed me to confront, on my own terms, years of accumulated mental, emotional, spiritual, and energetic dysfunction that had forced my body into pain, inflammation, fatigue, immobility, and isolation. Adding to my recovery have been recent medical breakthroughs in biological response modifiers and my introduction to Chinese herbs.

My energy has soared. I have been able to thrust myself with joy into my CranioSacral Therapy and physical therapy work, into bike trips and exercise, and into gatherings and relationships with friends and family.

Some might ask if I can tell whether it is the CranioSacral Therapy, the new medications, or the herbs that have been life-changing. I have played around with them all, allowing myself to get potentially lost by eliminating or decreasing one or the other over periods of time. What this has told me is that I need them all. Without CranioSacral Therapy or without medication or without proper nutrition and exercise, I still am prone to minor inflammatory flares.

I know there are parts of myself that still aren't sure how I can best be in this world. I feel that my body keeps me tuned into that. What I am sure of is that the scales have tipped. There are no longer huge amounts of old, negative emotion, blame, isolation, and distrust stuffed deep in my tissues. CranioSacral Therapy has allowed me to find my inner compass for the safe awareness and release of negativity and hurt. I can now easily get back to a home base within myself that feels hopeful and good. Pain and inflammation have peeled away in layers. For everything that helps me be at home in my body—CranioSacral Therapy being at the top of that list—I am extremely thankful.

Karen Jaeger, PT, CST
Madison, Wisconsin
CranioSacral Therapy Practitioner since 1993

Back on the Beat

One of my most memorable patients was a police officer who, during the course of apprehending a criminal, was rammed head-first into a wall before her partner arrived and seized the suspect.

Following this incident, Officer S★ began to have constant headaches. After several weeks of suffering increasingly incapacitating headaches, she was taken off her beat and placed on desk duty.

Before she was referred to our physical therapy clinic, Officer S had received no hands-on therapy. My time with her was limited to twenty- to thirty-minute sessions three times a week. My goal was to use only CranioSacral Therapy (CST) in her treatment.

After several weeks of CST, she reported a lessening of her headaches and dizziness. Then there was the unforgettable day when Officer S walked into the clinic with her uniform on and a big smile on her face. She had been reinstated to her beat! Several weeks later, she informed me that the sheriff had chosen her to be part of the department's very first bike patrol team.

This officer is now a detective and is continuing to do very well in her career. I feel very honored and blessed to have had a part in helping her by utilizing CranioSacral Therapy techniques.

Ellie O'Steen, LMT
Auburn, Alabama
CranioSacral Therapy Practitioner since 1987

★Name omitted to protect patient confidentiality

More Than a Stroke of Luck

❀ While attending Crystal Mountain Massage School in Albuquerque, New Mexico, I received a three-day introduction to CranioSacral Therapy (CST). During the first year in my own practice I occasionally used some of the simple diaphragm releases I had learned, although I felt nothing and questioned the validity of this technique.

Then one day a man called asking me to come to a private home to do CranioSacral Therapy on his sixty-eight-year-old father, Tom, who had suffered two strokes in the past month. He had heard that CST was good in these cases. I agreed to go to the home.

Tom's wife helped me get Tom out of his chair and onto the massage table. In my assessment I found Tom's right side to be totally affected by the stroke. To my surprise, he had equal energy in both legs.

After forty-five minutes of what felt like "going through the motions" on occipital and diaphragm releases, we got Tom off the table and back in his chair. They invited me to come back in four days for another session. When I returned, I got chills all over as Tom walked into the room on his own!

I made four visits to Tom's home in one month. On the last visit, he got out of his chair, walked down three steps without holding on, and climbed onto the table himself. My thoughts were: If CranioSacral Therapy can accomplish this from only a few techniques, I really ought to get some advanced training.

I believe this experience affected me and my practice as much as it did Tom. I have since completed CranioSacral Therapy level one, and it is now a regular part of my daily massage practice.

Jim French, LMT
Albuquerque, New Mexico
CranioSacral Therapy Practitioner since 2003

Bumps on the Head

CranioSacral Therapy (CST) has been very helpful in my own life, almost beyond description. My story, however, concerns my use of the technique on my wife.

Since she was a child, my wife has had two bumps on the top of her head. She experienced pain and pressure around these bumps, which caused headaches.

I decided to try CST to see if gently separating the parietal plates would relieve the area between the bumps, which it did. (The bumps were used as a reference point in knowing where to place the thumbs for the parietal work.) Right away the frequency of her headaches diminished, although she felt the same range of pain. As the sessions progressed, her pain intensity and headache frequency continued to lessen.

Today the compressed feeling around the bump region is gone. My wife continues to find CST very relieving for the region near the bumps. I often apply the therapy before she goes to sleep, which enables her to relax with a head of balanced movement and a mind in harmony with itself.

Winston Grace, LMT
Tamarac, Florida
CranioSacral Therapy Practitioner since 1997

Unwinding Brings Trauma Release

✿ A case that stands out is that of a husband and wife who drove twelve hours from another state for an appointment. The original appointment was for the husband. After I was done with him, I asked her if she wanted a session after all the time she had spent getting there. She refused several times but finally agreed after a lot of encouragement.

I gave the wife an intake form to fill out, but all she would put down was her name. Maybe she had some reason to be hostile, I thought. Using arcing techniques I was able to see that she had no pulse around the female organs, and her pulse was actually bound up inside her left shoulder. Releasing the long-time pain held in her left shoulder had the effect of restarting the pulse in the ovary area. At that point I felt that I was done for the day.

Three months later when the couple came through town I found out the rest of the story. First, she was an RN and didn't believe in this kind of work—hence her unwillingness to fill out the intake form. Second, for twenty-two years she had experienced increasingly painful monthly periods—painful to the point where she was missing a couple weeks of work each month.

As it turned out, the pain in this woman's shoulder was part of the pain from the birth of her now twenty-two-year-old son. After the single treatment, her periods had become pain-free. She received two more treatments after that, and I never saw her again.

Another client had experienced virtually continual migraines for eighteen years. When I met her, she had just come from her third hospital procedure where fluids were pumped in and out of the body in an attempt to stop the migraine cycle.

My first thought was: What happened eighteen years ago? Sure enough, there was a lot more to the story. A bad car accident had left her with half the skull missing, replaced by metal plates; her face and jaw bone reconstructed from other body bones; broken collarbones and ribs; and multiple knee surgeries. I had my work cut out for me.

After extensive CranioSacral Therapy, the headaches were better but hadn't stopped. I knew I was on the right road but was missing something. Unwinding the body through the many surgical operations, we discovered that she was pregnant when the accident occurred. The baby had been aborted to save her life, but she hadn't been given any say in the matter. We took the time for her to process the loss of her only child and to grieve for what had happened. Her incurable migraines of eighteen years stopped. She still had some sinus problems but not the migraines.

I saw this client twice a month for about nine months. She has since moved out of state.

John Carroll, RPP, CPT, RM
Lithonia, Georgia
CranioSacral Therapy Practitioner since 1997

CST Brings Renewed Life to Vietnam Veteran

The Imperial City of Hue, Republic of Vietnam, February 1968. It was relatively quiet on this side of the Perfume River. The heavy fighting was concentrated in the last holdout: the old Imperial palace known as the Citadel.

My platoon was in column formation, ready to move across one among the maze of streets that crisscross this beautiful city. I was in the middle of the column. The order came to move out. I was scared.

As the lead man started across the street, a sniper opened fire. The experience reminded me of a carnival; we were the mechanical cutouts passing in front of the sniper as he attempted to knock us down.

It came my turn to cross. I hesitated. My fear now fully in control of me, I motioned for the man behind me to go ahead. Then the next. I realized that I couldn't stay where I was, so I finally gathered myself together and made a mad dash for the far side of the street.

Pop! Snap! sounded the bullets as they flew unseen past me. I made it across the street unscathed, as did the rest of the column.

Ten months in Vietnam, and two more to go, if I lived. Ten months of energy-sapping fear, deprivation, mayhem, boredom, murderous heat and humidity, monsoon rains, biting insects, and exotic tropical diseases. Two more months of the sickly-sweet smell of human blood, the stench of burned flesh, the acrid smell of gunpowder, and the haunting memories of the screams of the wounded. It was all mind-numbing.

My hesitation in crossing the street that day in 1968, combined with other experiences, seeded a feeling of guilt in me that festered and grew for thirty-plus years. It became an aspect of what would, years later, be given the name post-traumatic stress disorder (PTSD).

In Vietnam we were forced into a state of highest possible alert, but we were never given the opportunity or knowledge of how to decompress our war experiences. We returned home as living time capsules, frozen in the memories of our tours of duty in Vietnam.

When and if we tried to find understanding through talking about our experiences, we found that few wished to hear about the horrors of what happened. Even to those who did lend a sympathetic ear, we found that our words were not adequate. How do you explain to someone what it really feels like to hold a close friend in your arms whose body has been horribly mangled and to hear his last words to you, hoarsely whispered, "Please don't let me die"? How do you admit to another and to yourself that you suspect the fear you felt while in Vietnam was actually cowardice? How do you share such profound feelings of grief, hopelessness, helplessness, inadequacy, and anger?

The answer is that you don't. Instead, you bury it all somewhere in your body and you shut down even further.

The PTSD Intensive Program for Vietnam Veterans that I participated in at The Upledger Institute HealthPlex clinic helped to restore my sense of hope, trust, and love. Through CranioSacral Therapy, SomatoEmotional Release, and the other approaches used at the clinic, I was finally able to begin speaking of my experiences. I realized that my memories were not just the imaginings of some crazed person. I saw that I was afraid to cross that street in Hue City not from a place of cowardice but from a place of sanity.

In one particular session we uncovered an aspect of me that was still hiding in abject fear and terror in a bunker somewhere in my unconscious mind. Letting this part of me know that the war was over was a most moving experience. I openly wept with profound relief from the absolute core of my being.

During the Intensive Program I felt I was finally heard; I opened to a deep healing in a roomful of dedicated beings who were able to love me unconditionally, even as I had been unable to love myself.

I believe that CranioSacral Therapy opened a pathway for my body to heal. I was so profoundly moved and inspired by the Cranio-

Sacral experience that I went on to train in the technique, and I hope to use it as I pursue a possible career of hands-on healing.

Roger Lansbury
Philadelphia, Pennsylvania
CranioSacral Therapy Practitioner since 2000

Connections and CST

✿ When I ponder how I have benefited from CranioSacral Therapy (CST), the word "connection" comes up over and over. The immediate therapeutic connection inherent in touch therapy is evident. The gradations of touch—from melding into tissue to light, energetic touch—give me varying hues of experience that are unique with each client.

My own personal connections with parts of myself I have either long forgotten or never known have altered significantly how I access the world. Life is no longer what happens to me, but is what I draw to myself. If I act out of fear, then I draw frightening situations towards me. Acting out of love by dropping into my heart brings compassion and love into my life.

I would have to say the type of connection that has been most profound is the connection I have experienced with people—specifically those who are drawn to CranioSacral Therapy as therapists. It is that connection I often think of and treasure.

I live and work in a small rural town in Michigan very similar to the small Indiana town where I grew up. Growing up on a farm in a large family afforded me the perspective of dreaming big while living simply. I have found that perspective shared by many people who live in a small, Midwest town atmosphere.

A few years ago I taught a one-day CST class developed by The Upledger Institute called ShareCare.® It was in that class I met Gerry. Like me, she dreamed big in her perceptions of what her life could be, but lived simply in a small Amish town in Northern Indiana. She had worked in a manual labor shipping business for over twenty-three years. Her visions of doing and being more brought her to the class and subsequently into my life.

Gerry's down-to-earth, practical, state-it-how-you-see-it approach took me back to the days before I received my higher education, which insisted on multisyllabic expressions of analysis.

That is not to say she couldn't keep up with the technical aspects of the work. In fact, she let words like "falx cerebelli," "superior sagittal sinus," and "occipital cranial base" roll off her tongue with a vivid description of what they are and what they do.

The connection Gerry made between where she was and where she needed to be came sometime during that class. Her confident touch connected with her compassionate heart and made it clear that her life was ready for a huge shift. And shift she did!

For the following year, Gerry juggled education in the Cranio-Sacral Therapy field with a full-time job. With absolute resolve, she enrolled in a massage school. She quit her job and joined a small bodywork practice in LaGrange, Indiana, serving much the same population as I do.

I believe this speaks to the truth and power in CST. Being a part of this simply dynamic therapy shows the potential transformation we can all have if we are open and willing. Big things can happen in very simple ways. Sometimes the process, once started, cannot be stopped. I found CST to be the ideal I needed to make that leap to becoming a bodywork therapist after years of being a psychotherapist. In fact, I have a tendency to think of my personal practice as a melding of my two areas of training. I often refer to my practice as somatic psychology.

Even with all of the in-depth education involved, I can't let go of the raw simplicity of CST—the touch, the intention, and the connection.

Gerry and I have kept in touch and see each other as often as our schedules allow. It can get lonely when one lives in a town we humbly refer to as "near nowhere." CranioSacral Therapy gave Gerry and me a connection that allows us to not only encourage each other but to grow as we share our insights about life with one another. Simply put, we continue to be the closest of friends. That I will cherish forever.

CST has led me to so many connections with people in this kind of practice who have experienced similar life transformations.

Those connections provide me the opportunity to continue to have faith in the process and connect with the energy of the universe that allows all creativity into being. That is the energy of connective intention.

Lauri Rowe, MA, CST-D
Coldwater, Michigan
CranioSacral Therapy Practitioner since 1998

CranioSacral Therapy and Animals

Blending is about melting and dissolving boundaries. Love is about blending.
—*John E. Upledger, DO, OMM*

Flashdancer's Story

❀ I met Flashdancer soon after her owner, Lisa, began to see me for CranioSacral Therapy sessions for her headaches and upper back and neck pain. Lisa and I were interested in how our lives had crossed, as she had been a Morgan horse breeder, and I had shown my two Morgan horses in upper-level dressage.

Lisa was surprised to hear that CranioSacral Therapy could also benefit horses and dogs. She told me the story of Flashdancer, her twenty-three-year-old mare, and asked if I might be able to help her.

Flashdancer is the alpha mare of Lisa's small group of horses. Two weeks previously, in the ice and snow of early spring, she took a severe fall in the pasture, her hind legs sliding out behind her. She was extremely stiff and had difficulty turning, especially in the confined quarters of her stall, pivoting on her front legs to try to shift her body.

Flash had also foundered about six months before the severe fall. The veterinarian suggested that her age, overweight condition, and insulin resistance had contributed to the painful inflammation in her hooves. Her founder had only partially resolved with the usual repeated, careful trimming of the hoof walls and special shoeing, as well as a homeopathic remedy.

Wanting some answers, Lisa consulted an animal communicator who told her that Flash could not even feel her hind legs and was afraid to walk on the ice. Flash told the animal communicator that she was very depressed after her fall and did not think she could continue to be the leader of Lisa's small herd of horses. She was very concerned about what would happen to her because she was unable to walk, or even stand comfortably. She reported to the animal communicator that she was not sure she could survive in so much pain and depression. Lisa had even seen the mare's hind legs buckle under her as she tried to make her way around the frozen pasture.

When I looked into her stall on a cold February day, Flashdancer was depressed and clearly in pain, shifting her weight between her feet to try to find a comfortable position. First, I introduced myself to this lovely, dark bay mare by gently allowing her to breathe in my scent as I exhaled close to her soft muzzle. I felt a deep respect for this horse instantly and could sense her long history of show-ring success and motherhood.

When I checked Flashdancer, I was drawn to her thoracic vertebrae and lower cervical area, with lesser involvement showing in her sacrum. As I recalled working with her owner, I realized that Flash had some of the same restrictions in her own body. When I told Lisa what I was finding, she was extremely sympathetic.

I spent an hour in our first session treating Flash's thoracic restrictions and dural tube, as well as working around her heart, all while Lisa told me what a good mother Flash had been for her foals. After I rebalanced Flash's sacrum, we could see that her hips were more level. Flash especially liked the tail-pull technique, and she leaned into my gentle resistance, giving herself a chiropractic treatment too.

At the end of the session, we could see Flash standing more balanced in her hind end, her hooves were both facing forward, and her expression was relaxed. I thanked her for working with me in the session, and she returned to her stall to rest.

After this first visit, Lisa reported that Flash was no longer stumbling with her back legs, and she had dramatically regained mobility. She was no longer pivoting around her front end to move her hindquarters. Lisa saw significant improvements in Flash's gait after the first session, and the mare seemed more comfortable standing in her stall.

I went to see Flash a second time about ten days later. She was much brighter and came to greet me when I opened her door. In this session, I focused more on her legs and hooves, using a regional tissue release technique on her hind legs and working on her temporal bones and poll (occiput in a horse).

Flash was very quiet during the session and seemed to know

that everyone was trying to help her. We could see the relaxation in the muscles in her thoracic area and even in her back above her kidneys. The muscles in her haunches were much more relaxed, and she was no longer hyperresponsive to light touches in her hamstrings and the insides of her hind legs. Lisa remarked that Flash's whole body looked more balanced after her second CranioSacral session.

After the second visit, the changes in Flashdancer were amazing. She began to jog to and from the field. She was back to her old self at feeding time, being frisky in her stall when she heard the grain buckets coming. Lisa saw her taking charge of the other horses in the field, rather than simply tolerating what was going on around her. Flash began to rear and stand on her hind legs in the pasture, plus trot and canter in the field. The farrier also reported better hoof growth after the two CranioSacral sessions, and Flash's founder is now completely resolved. She has lost some weight and looks much younger than her twenty-three years.

Incredibly, after a few more sessions with Lisa, we both noticed improvements in her upper-back restrictions and better approximation in her sacroiliac joints, which coincided with the improvements in Flashdancer. Although Lisa has not ridden Flash in many years, she is very connected to this horse. Some may say it is a coincidence that she and her horse had some of the same restrictions that improved simultaneously with CranioSacral Therapy. Lisa believes, however, that their journeys to wellness are as deeply intertwined as their love for one another.

Sally A. Morgan, PT, CST, TTEAM
Northampton, Massachusetts
CranioSacral Therapy Practitioner since 1994

CST Goes Wild

✿ Orca is a ten-year-old gray wolf who is a resident of Wolf Park, a research and education facility in Battle Ground, Indiana. As a young wolf, Orca was the alpha in his pack and had a reputation for "ruling with an iron paw," demanding submission of his pack mates to the point of being a tyrant. His submission technique was a hip slam that knocked his subordinate to the ground.

On November 27, 1997, Orca was found in his enclosure posed in a sphinx-like position. This kind of pose was not unusual; the fact that he was still in that position several hours later was.

Upon entering the enclosure, the staff found that Orca's hindquarters were paralyzed. He had sustained a spinal cord injury at L4 [lumbar vertebra] and had lost motor, sensory, bowel, and bladder function. A consulting vet advised euthanasia, but the staff elected to attempt rehabilitation.

Orca received medications, chiropractic intervention, massage, and acupressure over the next few months. Over time, Orca gradually regained use of his legs and function of his bowels and bladder. He remained weak, however, demonstrating a scissoring gait and frequent falls. He was also grumpy and out of sorts at times.

Enter CranioSacral Therapy (CST).

As a CST practitioner interested in Native American healing traditions, I have an interest in wolves and their reputation for being master healers and teachers. When a friend suggested that I visit a wolf sanctuary to learn more about them, I did a Web search, which led me to Wolf Park.

As I read Orca's story on their website, I thought, "This is a job for CST!"

I first met Orca in May of 2003. He was grumpy that day, so I visited with him from outside his pen. (No one goes in the pen with him when he is grumpy.) He was also eating, crunching through the ribs of his meal like they were candy canes. Although

I did not feel fear in his presence, the thought ran through my mind: "Maybe I should rethink this." Orca is a big fellow, and I noted that my whole head could easily fit into his mouth. Still I felt that we had an opportunity to make a difference in this wolf's life.

Veterinary approval was obtained, and Orca was offered CST for the first time on June 29, 2003. The staff advised me right away that Orca had declined all offers for help over the previous six months. So while they were willing to try CST, they clearly had little expectation for success.

Orca was invited over to me using hot dogs as enticement. Within a few minutes, he was standing and ready for work. I was astounded by what occurred. I had expected to spend a few minutes melding and evaluating him. He had other ideas.

Orca's dural tube began to elongate and release immediately when I placed my hands on him. He quickly took advantage of what was available and no longer needed hot dog invitations as incentive to come over and work. It was obvious to all who were observing that the CST made Orca feel good. The staff people were incredulous. "It looks like you aren't doing anything," they said.

Orca has continued receiving CST since that day. The intervals between sessions vary a great deal, depending on his mood and the availability of someone to treat him. (Staff members are being taught basic CST techniques.)

Orca has made improvement in his gait, endurance, and mood. After one of his sessions last summer, he was observed doing his "hop dance." He bowed, jumped in the air with a flip/twist, then landed and *ran* for a few steps around his enclosure. Tears welled up in my eyes when I was told that he hadn't been able to move like that since his injury.

Remember what I said about the wolf being a master healer and teacher? Orca is teaching thousands of others about Cranio-Sacral Therapy. His story and CST experience are on the park website. CST is discussed with park visitors when they inquire about Orca's health and recovery. And professionals from all over the world who study at Wolf Park are learning about CST. So not only is Orca an ambassador for his species, he is now an ambassador for CST. My life is forever changed by having the privilege of knowing and treating him. Orca's story will help change the lives of many others—human and nonhuman—by introducing them to CranioSacral Therapy.

Sandy Prantl, OTR/L, CST-D
Cincinnati, Ohio
CranioSacral Therapy Practitioner since 1992

It's Not Just for Humans Anymore

In October 2003, I decided to combine a love of horses with my therapy skills. I took some classes in equine CranioSacral Therapy (CST). I admit to starting my training feeling skeptical. How could such a light touch be effective on people, let alone creatures that are near, if not over, a thousand pounds? The transformations I have seen through the experiences of the horses receiving CranioSacral Therapy, however, are amazing and eye-opening.

Going into this work, I didn't know much about the logistics of horses; I still don't. What I learned over the past six months, though, is that horses are often treated with a heavy hand. They are subject to ego battles with their owners. They fight losing battles with dentists and veterinarians whose education deals in large part with medicating or operating. The horses have no voice in the matter, and the owners don't always know that other treatment options exist.

An old Indian legend tells how horses were not tamed by man. Horses volunteered to help man by letting him ride upon their backs and use them for work. Looking at this from a therapeutic context, I say the greatest beneficiary has not been the horse, but rather the man who administers the therapy to it.

Through a strange set of twists and turns, I find myself going to Long Island from Virginia Beach every few months to work on these great big clients. Sessions begin with a request to the horse for permission to work on him. Permission is then given to the horse to let go and heal.

Placing my hands gently on the skin (just lightly enough to imprint the fur) almost always brings a shocked reaction. As I alluded to previously, horses are not accustomed to such a light touch. New clients often will look back at me in amazement, as if to say, "When are you going to start doing something?" Or sometimes they glance back at me with a look of understanding, as if saying, "Oh, I get it, you're here to help; please go ahead." Then it begins to happen.

The horse, perhaps for the first time in a long while, begins to relax. The eyes droop. The lips become floppy. He may even drool! Almost always, if I place my hands on the body, the horse moves until my hands rest in the place that he feels needs the most attention.

During an equine CranioSacral Therapy session, we get very excited about signs of release—even gas! A big lesson here: Horses are very uninhibited in comparison to their human counterparts.

I have seen some dramatic changes in my clients. There were those that were too anxiety-ridden to be touched by strangers. For them, CST was a soft, reassuring hand letting them know that they could be touched without harm. There were those that were injured, and after three or so treatments showed less or no sign that an injury had even existed.

The biggest changes I have seen, however—bigger than the improvements in the equine clients—have been in the owners and how they relate to their horses. They can see that there are viable alternatives to surgery and medication—and not just for the horses. Many have asked to try CranioSacral Therapy. They are trying it, liking it, and spreading the word for humans *and* our four-legged companions.

Scott Warmbrand, CMT
Virginia Beach, Virginia
CranioSacral Therapy Practitioner since 2003

Freed from Fear

When I first met Amber, she had a splint on one of her rear legs and a cone collar on her head. She was shorn from the waist back, and there was a recent surgical scar on each hip. She was and is a beautiful dog—a red and white border collie the color of, well, amber. She was also not a very happy dog.

I was, among other roles in a busy life, a massage therapist, a student of CranioSacral Therapy (CST), and a volunteer foster home for Border Collie Rescue of California. Amber took one look at me and as much as said, "You're not going to touch me!"

She ignored the soft indoor quarters that I'd prepared for her, and instead established herself in one of the outdoor dog runs. She allowed me to walk her on a leash to do her business. When it came to bodywork, however, we sat in opposite ends of her six-foot-long dog run for the first two of our daily sessions.

I had just learned to work with the craniosacral rhythm off the body, in the energy field, and that is what we did in the beginning. The first time she pushed me out of her field. It was then that I tried freeze-dried liver, at which she turned up her nose. Then I tried peanut butter. She liked that.

On the third day, Amber allowed me to walk her around the house to the front porch, where she could see and hear the traffic yet feel protected. She did not like traffic. A few months earlier, she had escaped from her adopted family and been hit by a car. Her family found her by the roadside and paid for her extensive surgeries. They could not, however, deal with her special needs, so back she went to Border Collie Rescue. That's when I got her.

There on the front porch, Amber accepted CST and had her mysterious SomatoEmotional Releases, the contents of which only Amber knows for sure. She learned to back up to the corner of the porch and park her behind there. That way she wouldn't have to figure out what to do with her huge splint when she sat. Her neck and shoulders needed extensive work, as did her back. She always held her head high and back, in seemingly regal distaste for the world.

It was evident that Amber still had occasional panic attacks. After she could walk well on three legs and a splint, I often left her loose in the fenced yard, with my own dogs kenneled to prevent any possible roughhousing. One day something internal, external, or both prompted her to wedge herself (splint, cone, and all) between the fence and the chain-link dog run. She could not yet walk backwards, so we had to partially disassemble the dog run to free her.

Amber was with me for twenty-four days, until her vet appointments were completed. Then she went to one of the rescue kennels in the desert, where there was no traffic to vex her. After a few months, she got her own Web page and began interviewing prospective adopters. Following an extensive interview process, she eventually chose a woman with a large jar of peanut butter and an even larger heart. Amber and her new mom now walk on the sidewalk next to the cars, and they walk among strange people at Rescue and other events. We see each other at these events from time to time. In fact, only a few weeks ago, we were together at a Border Collie Rescue event. I was lying on the ground under a chair with Amber, releasing her sacrum.

Katherine Hutton, LMT
Pasadena, California
CranioSacral Therapy Practitioner since 2002

Crooked Bunny

It is not hard to miss a pen of bunnies at a horse show. After observing them for a few minutes with my friend, I realized that the head of one of them was severely twisted to the left. When she drank from the water bowl, she drooled a bit on the left side of her mouth. Her left ear lacked muscular development at the base; the weight of it was pulling heavily on her skull and other ear. She looked very uncomfortable and subdued, like a rabbit with a headache. She tried to support her head by snuggling up to her sleeping companions, resting her chin on their shoulders.

"Crooked Bunny," as she became known, was an adorable white rabbit with one slightly bluish eye and one brown, a small butterscotch spot on her nose, and a larger spot right over her sacrum. I raised rabbits for nearly twenty years, so I immediately felt compelled to help this little bunny.

I was told by the girl in charge that this eight-week-old bunny had simply been born crooked. Her head was tilted as a result of being in a big litter of eight; she hadn't had enough space to develop or move normally *in utero*. She agreed to let me work with the bunny during the show.

I held the bunny in my lap. It was unusually cold and rainy for July, so she gladly nuzzled in between my legs, resting her chin on my thigh. As I worked gently with two fingers of my left hand, I was pulled deeply through the fascia on her neck, until I could feel the side of the first cervical vertebra. Heat poured out of her neck as her head turned even further to the left at a crazy angle. The tissue held the position briefly, and then very slowly and surely it released, until minutes later her head was looking to the right for the first time in her short life. She then rolled onto her back in my hands and did a beautiful dural tube regional tissue release, which freed her entire spinal cord. It ended with a little kick from her hind feet as she turned herself right side up again.

For the rest of the session, I followed small releases in the bunny's head and neck as she closed her eyes and slept peacefully in my lap. When I had completed rebalancing of her sphenoid and sacrum, she opened her eyes, nibbled at my raincoat, and was ready to go back to the other bunnies. A model client, she relieved herself, drank a lot of water, did some grooming to smooth the fur on her head, and then settled in for a night's sleep next to her friends.

The next day, my friend who had been with me the day before called after stopping by the rabbit pen. She said, "The crooked bunny doesn't look so crooked anymore!" I arrived at the show and, sure enough, the rabbit had gained about fifty percent of normal cervical range of motion to the right, and her eyes seemed brighter.

As I knelt down, she hopped to the door of her pen and ran right into my hands. I could not have asked for a more clear sign of gratitude. This time, the CranioSacral Therapy focused over her left shoulder blade and the surrounding muscles, as well as on her temporal bones. She again dozed happily through the session, making small chewing sounds (a rabbit's form of purring). Her shoulder muscles were so tight and hot as the tissues released that I was surprised at her calm and trusting demeanor.

My dog, a corgi named Comet, took an interest in Crooked Bunny in the second session. He placed his nose gently on the butterscotch spot on her rump and held it there, stabilizing her sacrum and ilia, as I worked on her tiny temporal bones with one finger from each hand. She ended this session by licking Comet's cheek when she woke from her dozing.

On the third day, passersby were beginning to observe the CranioSacral sessions and commenting on how much better the bunny was moving her head. Comet continued to take part in the last three sessions, watching closely and then using his nose or a paw to assist me when he wanted to. The bunny acknowledged his help by licking him or purring when he contributed to the sessions.

By the fifth day, people could not tell which bunny had been the crooked one, though her head still had a slight tilt to the left. She was able to groom herself and seemed to delight in thoroughly cleaning the right side of her body. She drooled less when she drank and, most remarkably, seemed to have improved vision in the cloudy eye. She lacked good musculature in her left ear, but it did not pull her entire head to the left like before.

It was sad for Comet and me to say farewell to our friend, but I was assured that she was going to an excellent home with knowledgeable caretakers and older children to keep her company. "Not So Crooked Bunny" posed with Comet for some photos before I gently placed her on the ramp into the pen with her siblings one last time. As I released her, she paused and briefly touched my hand with her left forepaw, as if to say thank you before beginning the adventure of her new life.

Sally A. Morgan, PT, CST, TTEAM
Northampton, Massachusetts
CranioSacral Therapy Practitioner since 1994

Opening Gates

❀ Spirit Horse Ranch in Westcliffe, Colorado, is a center that offers support to people experiencing or ready to experience their own spiritual awakening and self-realization. The horses at the ranch play an integral role in this process. It is also home to donkeys, dogs (both four- and three-legged), and cats. During my stay there I had the opportunity to do CranioSacral Therapy (CST) with some of the horses. My afternoon with Bacardi was particularly memorable.

A handsome bay gelding, Bacardi had been with the owners of the ranch, Jill and Dave Eldredge, for over two years. Throughout that time, he had to be separated from the rest of the herd because of his behavior. He would prance and pace incessantly, thus upsetting the other animals. The dogs would become progressively agitated, and the other horses would drive him away.

My CST experience with Bacardi occurred mid-afternoon on a beautiful, bright, and clear February afternoon over a period of about two hours. I remember looking out across the vast, remote valley bordered by the huge, spectacular, snow-capped Sangre de Christo Mountains immediately to my left, and by the distant Wet Mountains to my right. A light blanket of snow covered the valley. Eight of the horses were together in one pasture while Bacardi and another gelding, Avatar, were separated in their own paddock.

As I stood watching the eight horses graze, I experienced a stillness unlike anything I'd ever experienced before. The herd felt so peaceful, and the horses seemed to be so present in the moment.

Bacardi, in contrast, seemed full of inner tension. I felt drawn to him and began to do some CranioSacral Therapy with him. As I placed my hands on his withers, I felt a sense of deep agitation and disconnectedness within him. He felt uncentered and ungrounded. Despite his apparent agitation, he voluntarily stood very still beneath my touch. As my hands explored his body I entered into a "soul-to-soul dialogue" with him. I told him what I was feeling and asked if his own inner wisdom would assist us.

I began treatment with a still point. (A still point is a time when the craniosacral rhythm stops. During this time the body is more able to release its restrictions and tensions and make its own self-corrections and adjustments.)

With Bacardi in still point, I encouraged him to connect with his own true self. Prior to coming to the ranch, he had been a show horse, and I talked with him about this. I wondered whether people had taught him to engage in behaviors that would make him stand out and be the "best." If so, were these competitive behaviors serving him well now? Were they appropriate for his life here on the ranch? I told Bacardi that I wanted to support him in whatever was in his highest good. It felt important that I work with him to facilitate an increased sense of his own centeredness and grounding.

The gates separating Bacardi from the rest of the herd had now been opened by Jill and Dave. Bacardi approached the other horses but kept a little distance. I stayed with him. He seemed to be following Avatar, the huge, stately black gelding who was his sole paddock mate. Avatar stopped and stood between Bacardi and the rest of the herd. Avatar's posture and presence seemed to provide a boundary to protect Bacardi from being chased off by the other horses.

As I continued the CST, Avatar and the donkeys looked on. It truly felt like these animals were holding sacred space for us. I could now feel Bacardi spontaneously going into his own still points, and it felt like he progressively quieted and settled into the core of his True Being. We stayed in that deep, quiet space together for a while, until it felt like Bacardi could sustain it by himself. I then took my hands off him and stood by his side. He remained calm and quiet. Then he turned his head toward me and nuzzled against my chest.

Bacardi proceeded to walk in to be closer to the other horses. He was able to remain calm in their presence for about ten to fifteen minutes. In the days that followed, he became progressively calm and centered. One by one, different horses would go over and "hang out" with him. Sometimes they would nuzzle him and show affection toward him.

Observing Bacardi over the next three weeks, I perceived that he was surrounded in love and support by all the two-, three-, and four-legged beings on the ranch. It was heart-warming to watch the progressive integration unfold.

It has now been four months since my CST session with Bacardi, and Jill writes the following:

"Since Veronica's visit, Bacardi has continued his process of integration within the larger Spirit Horse herd. Both he and Avatar now live with the rest of the horses twenty-four hours a day and are doing beautifully!

"I feel strongly that Veronica's support, skill, compassion, and presence absolutely helped him turn a corner that he simply couldn't negotiate on his own. He seems to have truly learned how to find his own 'still point' within. He remains the 'flightiest' of horses, but this is just a part of his own unique character, which he will probably always carry. However, he now has a way of working with his own intense energy that gently helps him to be a vital part of a herd that has always been just out of reach for him."

Veronica Quarry, MSPT
Arlington, Massachusetts
CranioSacral Therapy Practitioner since 1996

Spencer's Story

❀ Spencer was born on a beautiful, clear, warm fall day in September 2002. We had long anticipated and prepared for his birth—we just didn't know exactly when it was to happen. You see, Spencer is an alpaca, which is in the llama family. They tend to be smaller than llamas and are prized for their fleece.

At first Spencer appeared okay, just a little slow and quiet. His lovely, soft, cinnamon-colored hair complemented his deep-brown, sleepy eyes. After a few days, though, it became clear that something was not quite right. Spencer could not lift his long neck or support his head upright. When he tried to stand and nurse, his rear legs would buckle under him and he would fall over. Once on the ground Spencer would rarely try to get up again.

Examinations by a veterinarian and even an alpaca specialist yielded no clear diagnosis and no real plan for treatment. "Everything seems normal," they said. "He must have 'failure to thrive'; there is not much we can do."

By his tenth day, Spencer was being fed goats' milk through a tube. He received saline injections because he was so dehydrated. This treatment soon gave him strength enough to stand, albeit wobbly.

Within a couple of weeks he was doing a better job of nursing. But Spencer was still unable to lift his head. He would walk around tethered to his mother, his nose on the ground like a bloodhound hot on the trail of an escaped convict. Normally, when alpacas sit or "cush" on the ground, they hold their heads upright atop their long, strong necks. Poor Spencer could only lie down with his head flat out in front of him. He never interacted or played with the other alpacas or llamas. He seemed sad and alone.

That is when I got the call, at the beginning of Spencer's third week. His human mother, Lisi, is a patient of mine. In my practice as a naturopathic physician and acupuncturist, I perform Cranio-

Sacral Therapy, which I learned from The Upledger Institute. I have been incorporating it into my practice for more than ten years. Lisi hoped my training could help Spencer.

As I watched Spencer walk around the yard during my first visit, I noticed that the movement of his hindquarters was greatly restricted. His hind legs were scooted under him, and his sacral area and low back had no fluidity of movement. His back legs did not seem to work independently. His head was held low and did not rise even as I approached.

Lisi and I got Spencer into a sitting position, and I placed my hand on his sacrum. It was locked in flexion with no movement whatsoever. There were corresponding restrictions in his back at the fascia interface between the upper thoracic and the neck. The base of his skull felt jammed onto his vertebrae. He had very little cranial rhythm. Spencer did not display the normal inquisitiveness of a young alpaca. Instead of sniffing me out, he would just lie there on the ground as though his short life had already been a long and weary one.

Because the veterinarian had ruled out any pathology or disease process, I believed that a birth trauma was the most likely cause of Spencer's symptom picture. My initial goal was to release some of the restrictions in the sacrum. Along with using CranioSacral Therapy to enhance the flexion and extension of the sacrum, I used some acupressure points along the lateral edge of the sacrum. With each response in his sacral rhythm, and with each softening of the restrictions, Spencer would inhale fully and let out a big sigh of relief. I worked with Spencer for about twenty minutes, releasing restrictions in his sacrum, neck, and occiput.

After this first session, Spencer was able to bring his head up parallel to the ground—a big improvement over the "vacuum cleaner" pose that his head had been in for the first month of his life! He still made scooty little steps when he walked, but his hind legs were beginning to move independently and his balance was better.

Over the course of the next few weeks, I worked with Spencer four times. Each time I visited, he would eye me cautiously from across the yard, scamper away, and then come closer to check me out. This interaction went on for a few minutes. He would soon cush, and I would sit over him. He seemed to enjoy the contact. With each session, as his cranial rhythm improved, he improved. Quite noticeably he began to hold his head upright. Before long he could nurse without falling over, and his rear legs moved freely.

By the fourth session, Spencer was acting like any other six-week-old alpaca. He was alert, active, and playing with abandon and vigor!

With the gift of CranioSacral Therapy, I was able to help Spencer recover from a birth trauma that would have, in all likelihood, prevented him from living through his first winter.

Now nearly two years old, Spencer is active and rambunctious, giving great joy to all those who know him. That in and of itself is payment enough for me. Yet nothing quite beats the soft comfort of the beautiful cinnamon-colored sweater that I wear with great fondness when the warm days of fall give way to the cold winds of winter.

Steve Stroud, ND
Wenatchee, Washington
CranioSacral Therapy Practitioner since 1992

Major—The Oldest Great Pyrennees

✿ When I looked into his deep-brown eyes three years ago, I could see that Major was a wise old soul. The calm and peace in his gaze said that he had seen and understood many things in his lifetime. Major was twelve years old then, a huge, white, fluffy Great Pyrennees. Just back from the groomer, he had a tiny blue bow on his collar.

After we exchanged greetings, Amy, his owner, told me about Major's past. He had worked on a llama ranch in Minnesota as a guard dog, but he kept running away. He was adopted by a young vet student and acclimated to living indoors. He was difficult to manage and very possessive of her, however, which proved too challenging when she later married.

Still recovering from the death of her German shepherd, Amy offered to be a foster home for Major when he was turned over to Pyrennees Rescue at the age of nearly eight years. Major had a history of severe separation anxiety, but when she brought him to her house, he walked in, settled down, and clearly felt like he had finally come home. Amy knew immediately that Major was to become her constant companion for the rest of his life.

Amy had recently found out that her beloved companion had laryngeal paralysis. Often seen in older animals, it affects the opening to the airway in the throat, making it easy for them to inhale food into their lungs. Surgery is usually recommended to tie open the airway for improved breathing; however, this also makes it even easier for food to be inhaled into the lungs, resulting in pneumonia and possible death. The prognosis can be poor even after the surgery, so Amy was anxious to try all possibilities before deciding on surgery. A friend whose boxer I had helped recommended that she bring Major to me for CranioSacral Therapy (CST).

Despite his condition, Major still got up to bark, albeit hoarsely, when someone came to the door. Amy loved Major's booming baritone bark and was very sad to think that his laryngeal paralysis might make it impossible for him to bark at all.

Major also was quite arthritic, showing stiffness in his hind end and struggling with incontinence. He made some attempts to be in charge of Amy's other dogs and cats, but his general demeanor was listless when I met him.

As soon as I placed my hand on his huge head, Major relaxed and lay down on his rug. My hands felt deeply pulled into the bones in his head and the tissues underneath. I worked a lot on his neck and hyoid muscles, freeing up many restrictions where his skull connected to his first neck vertebra.

Major was in a very sound sleep for most of his first treatment. He stirred occasionally to yawn or shift his body position. I finished the session with some work on his sacrum and dural tube, rebalancing the relationship between his skull bones and his sacrum. I did not want to disturb him, so I left quietly, wondering what would come from his first CranioSacral Therapy session.

Amy called me two days later to report that her partner had noticed a huge change in Major. "He's acting like a puppy," he told her excitedly. Major was pulling on his leash during his walk, trotting up the big hill to the woods behind their house. "I could barely hold him back," Amy's partner said.

Major was much more animated around the house, interacting more with the other dogs and cats. A relief to Amy, he was no longer having such intractable incontinence. He was guarding his bones from the other dogs and was very feisty—he was back to his old self. Amy reported that Major was no longer gasping for air and panting continuously. "He's barking again!" she said. "I thought I had heard that bark for the last time."

I have continued to see Major for CranioSacral Therapy for the past three years. In the early months of his treatments, Amy noticed that he would become depressed and limp more on his walks if too much time passed between sessions.

I now see him about two times a month. Amy notices that after a day of sleeping following a session, he seems rejuvenated, plays more, and goes back to his job of barking to alert everyone in the house about visitors. She also sees improvement in his bowel and bladder control after his sessions, and he seems to be doing quite well cognitively.

Amy has added some small dogs to her family, and Major is a benevolent caretaker overseeing their puppy antics. He has some stiffness in his gait but still enjoys his walks.

Large dog breeds, like the Great Pyrennees, are often expected to live about nine years, so Amy was initially cautious in giving too much of herself to a dog already considered elderly at eight.

I thought I was coming into Major's and Amy's lives to ease his transition out of this life. Instead, I have now known Major for three years. He celebrated his fifteenth birthday on March 28, 2004, and he continues to do well. Thanks to CranioSacral Therapy, Amy and her beloved companion have shared many more years together than she had thought possible when they first met.

Sally A. Morgan, PT, CST, TTEAM
Northampton, Massachusetts
CranioSacral Therapy Practitioner since 1994

The Healing of My Furry Friend

✻ I took my first CranioSacral Therapy (CST) class in the spring of 2003. My full-time job at that time was Director of Rehabilitation Services for a pediatric health system in New Jersey. I had been interested, however, in holistic healing since the mid-eighties and had trained in Reiki, massage, hypnotherapy, and other modalities, which I utilized mainly for family. After this CST class, I was inspired to move toward my dream of holistic healing as my career.

To say that my experience with CST has been life-changing would be an understatement. I am still Director of Rehab, but only part-time. In my CST practice, I see approximately twenty-five clients. Incredible things occur during almost every session. There is one client story, however, that is exceptionally special and different from all the rest.

Peaches is a fifteen-year-old Bijon/Maltese mixed breed under veterinary care for congestive heart failure. She lives across the street from me.

Her "mother," Sharon, called me one evening stating that Peaches had hurt her leg. She wanted to know if I would "do that thing you do" for her. Of course the answer was yes.

Initial evaluation revealed an inability to bear any weight on the right hind leg; an extremely asymmetrical and jagged craniosacral rhythm; and significant weakness and decreased amplitude to the right during flexion. I began with a still point induction, which she responded to very quickly and maintained for several minutes. Direction of energy (applied hip-paw) resulted in multiple therapeutic pulses and marked heat release.

According to Sharon, Peaches didn't take to most people and didn't like to be touched for any length of time. She appeared quite content, however, as she snuggled up against me throughout the session. Peaches truly seemed to be "soaking it up," turning her head periodically to lick my hand as if saying thank you.

Interestingly, just as I would intend to change my hand position to facilitate a diaphragm release, she would reposition herself in just the needed way. Direction of energy and CV-4 techniques were done between diaphragm releases, with continued heat release and therapeutic pulsing observed. During the pelvic diaphragm release, my hands appeared to actually meld with Peaches—first one, then the other, then both.

The session lasted approximately fifty minutes. Upon completion, Peaches stood up and attempted to walk. Granted, her leg remained very weak, with repeated collapsing, but still an incredible improvement had occurred from baseline.

Peaches received five shorter follow-up sessions over the next few weeks. Each time she walked up to me as if ready and eager to begin. At that point complete recovery of function had occurred. Although that alone is a wonderful story, there is much more.

Three months later, during a regular checkup, Peaches' veterinarian commented that her cardiac function was "looking really good." But then, just over a month later, the dog lost all function on her left side. She could not walk, stand up, or relieve herself without assistance. She was rushed to University of Pennsylvania Veterinary Hospital in Philadelphia. The neurologist gave possible diagnoses of either a very fast-growing brain tumor with no hope of recovery, or a stroke with limited prognosis due to her age. As a result, Sharon and husband Lou were giving serious consideration to euthanasia.

Sharon called me, and that evening I worked with Peaches, utilizing direction of energy to the cranial vault (occipital, frontal, temporal, parietal bones), diaphragm releases, and multiple still points. Initial arcing pointed to the right side of the occipital base. The craniosacral rhythm was almost unpalpable on the right, and there was a strong sense that the source of the hemiplegia was not of a progressive nature. The session lasted over an hour and felt extremely deep, as though Peaches were engaged in healing from her very core.

After two thirty-minute follow-up sessions that week, Peaches was able to bear weight on the affected side. She then received CST twice weekly over the next several weeks. By month's end, she was walking, though some residual paresis of her left front leg/paw was noted. In addition, she was not yet able to successfully handle changes in elevation (e.g. single step, bumpy ground).

All sessions were approximately twenty to thirty minutes in length and consisted primarily of multiple still points, direction of energy, and diaphragm releases. Peaches consistently evidenced therapeutic pulses, heat, and respiratory changes as signs of release of membranous restrictions and healing. Six months into treatment, Peaches successfully climbed single steps and was attempting the stairs to the second story. Thirty-nine days post-stroke, I received an elated call: Peaches had climbed the full flight of stairs, pausing at the top to bark for attention and praise for her incredible feat! Needless to say, we were all literally thrilled to tears.

I still give Peaches an occasional "boost," especially prior to her visits to the groomer. Sharon reports that Peaches' previous anxiety is greatly reduced, especially important given her heart condition.

There really does appear to be more pep in Peaches' step now, and, as Sharon says, "My fifteen-year-old dog acts like a puppy again." I personally feel truly blessed to have been a part of my little friend's amazing recovery. Thank you, Dr. John, and Upledger Institute.

Janet Hensenne-Rosiak
Sicklerville, New Jersey
CranioSacral Therapy Practitioner since 2003

The Cat Who Fell from a Tree

❀ Bebe Kitten's story began when she was taken home from the SPCA (Society for the Prevention of Cruelty to Animals). Within months, she was shivering in the snow, ice balls in her long, fluffy fur.

Ann had seen Bebe thrown outside like she was a bag of rubbish. Taking her in, she called her daughter Mickey, who had been wanting a cat. Delivered to her new home, Bebe settled in.

She was a tiny cat, weighing five pounds at most. A fluffy, long-haired calico, Bebe spent evenings basking by the fire, dozing on the sofa, or lying on the lap of Mickey's husband Barry. In summer, she spent lazy afternoons sleeping in the sunshine in the wicker chair on the porch. While she could come and go from the house as she pleased, she never strayed more than ten feet from the yard surrounding her cottage home. She had two full meals a day and invitations to share the bed with her parents.

Bebe Kitten was my neighbor. I passed by her lookout on her porch chair every day when I went to walk my dog on the path that ran by her house. When Mickey called to say that something terrible had happened to Bebe, I went to their house immediately.

Bebe was crouched on the floor, hiding near the fireplace, mewing in distress and pain. She had not eaten in a day and a half. The visiting veterinarian who examined her said that Bebe had dislocated her patella (comparable to the human knee) and would require surgery immediately at great expense.

Uncertain what to do considering the high cost of the surgery, Mickey asked for my opinion. I said I'd like to try CranioSacral Therapy, as the injury was very recent. Perhaps we could more clearly see what to do after the session.

Bebe protested in pain when Barry gently lifted her onto his lap. Initially I could not even touch the painful side of her hindquarters, so I worked with one hand over her left uninjured hip and the other just barely touching the fluff over her painful joint.

Heat poured out from the injury as the tissue began the release process. Bebe was very uncomfortable at the beginning of the work. She meowed loudly and squirmed. Sensing that we were trying to help her, however, she made no attempts to get away. Gradually I was able to release enough trauma around Bebe's patella joint to be able to work specifically on the injured tendons and ligaments using just two fingertips on her tiny body.

By the time the session progressed to regional tissue release on her right hind leg, Bebe was purring and sleeping, trusting us not to hurt her. It felt like she had experienced a sudden concussion on the hind leg that had led to her injuries. I followed her hind limb as it moved through what seemed to be her protective limping and struggle to return to the safety of her spot by the fireplace.

While I finished with some dural tube work and sacral rebalancing, I explained to Mickey and Barry that Bebe would rest for a very long time after the session. I instructed them to put food and water right next to the soft bed they had ready for her. I also suggested putting the clean litter box right near the bed so she would not have to move very far for the twenty-four hours.

The next evening when I got home from work, Mickey came to meet me at my car. She said, "She did exactly what you said she would. She slept for almost twenty-four hours. Then she got up, used her box, stretched, and walked over to ask Barry to put her on the sofa. She even ate her dinner!"

I went with Mickey to see Bebe Kitten. Barry held her again as I checked her hind leg. This time she began to purr and snore right away as I worked over her pelvic diaphragm and then more directly over her patella. While the first session lasted over an hour, this session was only fifteen minutes long. I knew Bebe had gotten what she needed when she opened her sleepy eyes, looked up at me, and then delicately licked my hand as if to say thank you.

Bebe did not need to have surgery. She made a full recovery by the end of the week. We found out later that a neighbor had seen her fall out of a small apple tree next to her house. That explains why I had sensed a concussive force through her right hind leg during the regional tissue release work.

Bebe has shown no difficulty walking or jumping in the four years since I treated her. At fifteen years old, she is still happily passing the afternoons sunning in her rocking chair on the porch, and the evenings curled up with Barry and Mickey on the sofa by the fireplace.

Sally A. Morgan, PT, CST, TTEAM
Northampton, Massachusetts
CranioSacral Therapy Practitioner since 1994

Index

Contact Information

For information on healthcare continuing education workshops for professionals and educational materials (modalities include CranioSacral Therapy, SomatoEmotional Release®, Visceral Manipulation, Lymph Drainage Therapy, Healing From the Core, and related techniques):

The Upledger Institute, Inc.®
11211 Prosperity Farms Road D-325
Palm Beach Gardens, Florida 33410-3487

Phone: 1-800-233-5880 or 561-622-4334
Fax: 561-622-4771

Website: www.upledger.com
E-mail: upledger@upledger.com